EFFECTIVE INTERACTION IN CONTEMPORARY NURSING

EFFECTIVE INTERACTION IN CONTEMPORARY NURSING

CHARLOTTE EPSTEIN
Temple University

PRENTICE-HALL, INC., Englewood Cliffs, New Jersey

Library of Congress Cataloging in Publication Data

EPSTEIN, CHARLOTTE.
   Effective interaction in contemporary nursing.

   1. Nurses and nursing—Psychological aspects.
   2. Nurse and patient. I. Title. [DNLM: 1. Nurse-patient relations. 2. Nursing.
WY87 E65n 1974]
RT86.E67   610.73'019   73-7857
ISBN 0-13-241448-1
ISBN 0-13-241430-9 (pbk.)

Printed in the United States of America

10 9 8 7 6 5 4 3 2 1

Prentice-Hall International, Inc., *London*
Prentice-Hall of Australia, Pty. Ltd., *Sydney*
Prentice-Hall of Canada, Ltd., *Toronto*
Prentice-Hall of India Private Limited, *New Delhi*
Prentice-Hall of Japan, Inc., *Tokyo*

For Ralphie—

driven to do his learning the hard way

CONTENTS

PREFACE

In the world today, people are searching for themselves. They are struggling to discover their essential humanity in the morass of pollution, racism, war, and poverty. Sensitivity training sessions and confrontation groups proliferate. College courses in group dynamics and human relations are oversubscribed. The "free" high schools and universities offer opportunities to question everything we have heretofore accepted as a society and on which we have built our lives.

Slowly and painfully we are beginning to see ourselves in relation to one another, to touch one another, and to express our feelings about ourselves and the people near us. There is a revolution going on, and the revolution is rooted in our growing appreciation of our own humanness.

It is not surprising that the dynamic, exciting, and frightening processes of change we are experiencing in the world should be mirrored in the nursing profession. For nursing is at the heart of the action. In an area where concern with life and death, poverty and affluence, knowledge and ignorance, and feelings and intellect converge in some of the most basic human relationships, the nurse is one of the important people involved.

Nurses are struggling today to make use of what we have learned and continue to learn about human relationships. Perhaps more than any other profession, nursing is faced with the necessity of redefining professional roles and reassessing traditional professional values. This reassessment ranges all the way from planning to become deliverers of primary health care to considering whether or not the nurse's cap and uniform should be discarded.

Out of the struggle, the nurse will inevitably emerge, I think, as the leader of the health team; because in the person and function of the nurse will come together the scientific knowledge, the practitioner's skill, the information and skills and sensitivities needed for effective human interaction—and the ability to articulate the means and ends for optimum health care in our society.

It is nurses who are studying human relations. It is nurses who are—as a profession—trying to come to terms with a society's fear of death and its rejection of the aged. It is nurses who are risking themselves to develop skills for working in teams: risking themselves by expressing their feelings and opinions, taking firm stands on professional issues, and encouraging participation of personnel traditionally exluded from the health team. This is not to say that people in other professions are not doing many of these same things. But it seems to me that the commitment *as a profession* to human relations is more prevalent and pervasive in nursing than elsewhere in the healing and service professions.

This book is designed primarily for nurses—those who are preparing for nursing and those who have been nursing for years and are now caught up in the new dynamics of change. The methods and techniques for becoming actively involved in the process of self-examination, education, and change are described here in ways, I hope, that are practical and useful. Hundreds of nurses at all levels of the process have tried these methods and have contributed to their modification. The techniques work for those who are willing to try them.

Let the nursing instructors lend themselves to the processes, joining their students in the risky business of talking about their feelings and practicing interactive skills. The relationships that result from the teaching-learning situation can be models for nurse-patient relationships. After all, can we maintain that the nurse-patient relationship should be less open, less warm, less satisfying, less productive than the nurse-nurse relationship?

C.E.
Philadelphia

EFFECTIVE
INTERACTION
IN
CONTEMPORARY
NURSING

1 *WHAT NURSES WANT TO KNOW*

EXPRESSING CONCERNS: COOPERATIVE PLANNING

Students come to any teacher filled with questions, torn with anxieties, perplexed with problems, alternately eager and fearful of what the new term will bring. Why, then, do they sit back in their seats, open their notebooks, and indicate by their posture and expression that it is all up to the teacher? After all, they are the ones who have chosen to be nurses. Presumably they have some ideas about what is involved in such a choice. Why, then, do they seem to be saying that they have nothing to contribute to their own professional education? Why do they give the impression that they are merely receptacles, waiting for the knowledge that is shortly to be poured into them by the authority in front of the room?

Generally, the experience of students has been that teachers—from kindergarten through the university—are prepared with plans, courses of study, and curricula that leave little room for students' suggestions. Not only do teachers imply that they know exactly what students need, but they are often harried and concerned because there is not enough time to "cover" everything that has been designated as "required." In the last rush of class sessions before examinations, it is not unusual for instructors to speed up the pace of their lecturing and to request that the students refrain from asking questions, so that all the material may be presented before the end of the term.

The dutiful students take their notes more quickly, cram diligently for examinations, and then go on to the hospital floor to be told by graduate nurses that what they are learning in school is so much nonsense, because "here we do things entirely different." So much for covering the course of study!

Perhaps I am overstating the case, but there are some important issues to be considered here: (1) How much of any course of study do students remember ten weeks after the end of the course? (2) How much of the material in a course is "required" only because it has always been required? (3) How are learning and behavior affected by ignoring the concerns of students? (4) And how does all of this affect the future of the nursing profession?

There is enough evidence in the field of learning to convince even the most die-hard dispenser of information that most of what students learn through lectures is very quickly forgotten. Unless the information is almost immediately put to use in some meaningful way, there does not seem to be much point in reciting reams of facts and observations to large groups of note-takers. If the lecturer completes a semester with a feeling of satisfaction because she has given all the lectures she had planned and the students have done fairly well in repeating the information on examination papers, she is deluding herself. There really is no evidence that examination grades predict effectiveness in nursing. We know this, yet most of us are unable to make the break from those traditional teaching methods that, at the very least, make education dull for most students.

Maybe the primary difficulty is that we simply have nothing with which to replace the old methods. Who has ever taught us to use the available alternatives? Even students of education—if they are exposed to alternative methods of teaching at all—only hear about them in lectures and read about them in books. Their professors rarely teach them by methods other than lecturing.

Nursing educators may maintain that what the students get in lectures they immediately put to use in clinical practice, and so the lecture material is reinforced in the practical setting. I doubt that this is any more true of nursing that it is of education or law. Most of the information given in lectures is not immediately related to clinical practice. If it does have any value for professional functioning in the long run, then we need to help students learn it in ways that will help them to retain it. Lectures are the least efficient way to ensure that learning will be retained.

But are the traditional bodies of knowledge really important in the professional education of nurses, or are many included only because they have always been included? I am certainly not the one to answer this question. I can only raise it. And I feel confident that it needs to be thought about because I see similar situations in other professions. I recall the liberal arts professor who seriously contended that the courses required for the liberal arts degree were determined in the eighteenth century for good and valid reasons. The reasons, he assured me, were as valid today. Three centuries of accumulated knowledge, three centuries of changing political structures and social expectations, three centuries of values discarded and replaced, had apparently not affected his approach to the education of students!

Perhaps the most important question that all of us in education must ask ourselves is: What is the effect on learning and behavior of imposing traditional courses of study and ignoring the concerns of students? One of the consequences I have seen over and over again is a mounting frustration and anxiety that often explodes into outright rebellion. When that happens, *everything* in the program is rejected out of hand, instructors are scathingly attacked for everything that they do and say, and almost all learning stops for large blocks of time until feelings subside somewhat—only to rise again at the next crisis. All this is an obvious waste of energy and time, to say nothing of the toll it takes in eroding human relationships. Although some program directors maintain that the recurrent crisis is "normal," I regard this as an excuse for not looking at the causes and cures.

When the acute and persistent pressure to work toward pre-set objectives and to produce grades on examinations is removed, these emotional group crises do not occur. And, contrary to the fears of teachers, the quality of the students' work does *not* deteriorate. Although it is true that some students do not work unless pressured, it is also true that some students who *are* pressured do not work. However, in the free and open educational situation, students who do not work will eventually "de-select" themselves. In the traditional program, too many students make a game of getting away with it. And they often succeed.

Many nursing educators bemoan the persisting rigidity of nursing education and practice. As in most other institutionalized professions, change is slow and painful, and the quality of human relationships seriously interferes with optimum professional practice. As long as the practitioners of a profession are educated in situations and by methods that encourage rigidity and as long as they ignore human relations education, then the profession is stacking the deck against itself and fostering its own resistance to change.

Those of us who are engaged in teaching, no matter what body of data we are teaching, have been given the word by students: They will no longer accept what we give them without questioning, voicing their doubts, and resisting our fiats. They are much too caught up in the anxieties and excitements of a rapidly changing world. Contemporary events are closing in on them and they demand a share in shaping their own destinies. Nor are they willing to consider their time in school as some kind of preparation for life. School *is* their life now and they want to live it actively. What *they* think, what *they* believe, what *they* feel must be considered in defining school objectives and experiences, or we will lose the best of them to trial-and-error experimentation with alternate life styles.

This does not mean that there are not many students who seem perfectly willing to continue their passive, conformist educations. They have been well trained by their teachers in elementary and high school. But we must not see this passivity as satisfaction nor this conformity as contentment. It is merely a conditioned response that dulls creativity and breeds resignation.

There are techniques for encouraging students to express their concerns and for incorporating them into the process of curriculum development. These methods and techniques help students develop self-actualizing modes of behavior and make their human relationships more satisfying. All of this contributes to their ability to learn the technical knowledge and skills of their profession and then go on to make their personal and professional lives more dynamic and productive.

One way to encourage students to participate actively in the teaching-learning process is for the instructor to make it clear that the students' contributions are valuable. Generally, we think we are conveying this attitude when we say "that's right" or "that's good" or "I agree" when a student answers a direct question. And then we go on to elaborate *our own* original thought. There is little in this approach that really convinces the student that he is contributing anything to the subject. It is more like being patted on the head and simply reinforces student dependence on teacher evaluations and approval.

However, to take a student's response and use it, building on it and encouraging other students to do the same, is to make the students *know* that they are reaching beyond the instructor's question and drawing on their own knowledge and awareness. Thus, the instructor starts by asking: "What do you want to know about nurse-patient relations?" Since the student is the best judge of what he *wants,* there is really no necessity for any teacher comment at this point. The job of the teacher is merely to record all the student responses and then use them as a basis for teaching the course in nurse-patient relations.

If you are not enrolled in a formal course of study but are merely meeting as a group of professionals to add to your information, sharpen your sensitivity, and refine your skills, then the same principle applies. As a group you are concerned about certain matters involving the relations between patients and nurses. The first task is to get as many of these concerns as possible out in the open and recorded so that you can proceed to address yourselves to those concerns.

There is an advantage in answering the question aloud and writing the responses down verbatim. Individuals who are usually reluctant to speak out in a group need not feel threatened by a teacher's or leader's evaluation of their response. People who have never put certain of their concerns into words are encouraged to say what they feel when they hear other people speaking up. The group becomes aware of the wide range of issues that concerns their colleagues. Not the least advantageous of listing these concerns and then dealing with them in an educational situation is the assurance that you are dealing with matters that are interesting and important to the students or participants. It gets one away from the tired old programming under which an institution makes all the decisions about what is needed by every student and professional who passes through its doors.

The teacher who uses this technique to develop a course of study discovers that most of the topics she considers important are considered important by her students, too. As the class deals with topic after topic, their perceptions of the field become broader and more sophisticated. After five or six weeks of study, if they are asked the question again: *"Now, what do you want to know about nurse-patient relations?"* the responses will reflect a higher level of knowledge and sensitivity. Thus the teacher— or group leader—can diagnose the effectiveness of the learning situation and make some judgment about what the students are missing. In this way the teacher need never worry that what she is contributing to a course is inadequate. In her role as diagnostician, facilitator, and resource person, she is much more likely to produce educated professionals than she did when she served up facts and then read those same facts handed back to her on examination papers.

This census technique not only gives students the opportunity to study what they are interested in, but also represents a good first step in cooperative curriculum planning, good for the instructor as well as the students. The instructor who has grave doubts about students being any- thing but recipients in the teaching-learning process is very quickly con- vinced that students are more able, more knowledgeable, and more *serious* about the requirements of professional education than they are ever given credit for.

The technique is not very difficult, but it does have some pitfalls that must be avoided if it is to work.[1]

> 1. The question asked must be broad enough so that everyone can offer a response, and narrow enough so that the total response can be used as the unit or the course.
>
> 2. The original question must not be altered in order to encourage more responses.
>
> 3. Every response must be used in planning the unit or the course.

[1] See my book, *Affective Subjects in the Classroom: Exploring Race, Sex, and Drugs* (Intext, Scranton, Penna., 1972) for a detailed description of this and other teaching techniques.

4. The teacher must refrain from evaluating the students' responses and must discourage such evaluation by other students. In other words, every response is "right" and must be treated as equal in importance to every other response. It must be recorded verbatim, with no attempt to change the student's wording.

If the student is convinced that the course really will deal with his concerns and interests, and that every contribution will not immediately be evaluated, he is encouraged to lend himself more actively to the planning process and, subsequently, to the total process of learning. The wariness and even fear that so many students feel in the classroom, feelings that make them play it safe by merely doing what the teacher wants them to do, eventually may be somewhat dispelled.

When the census has been completed, the students should be assured that, if another question or topic occurs to them, they will be free to add it to the list. Then it is time to take the items in the census and begin to make decisions about how to deal with each item.

ONE HUNDRED CONCERNS

In one class of fifty third-year students in a baccalaureate program (their first year of nursing), I asked the question: "What do you want to know about nurse-patient relationships?" These are the responses that poured out of the students:

Professionalism. What it means and what is the purpose of it?

How far do you place your personal likes and dislikes on to the patient?

Why the frustrations that seem to be obvious among nurses and very directly affect how they come across?

Patient's attitude toward nurse as a babysitter, maid, housekeeper, not as important as the doctor. (That's true, I think.)

How about priorities to task orientation—humanitarianism?

Myths of sterotypes.

Psychological end, as far as the nurse is concerned. What she should say to the patient and how.

How would you deal with a criminal that's been shot or something?

How can we deal with sexism?

If a member of your family is a patient on the floor, is it possible to be detached?

What are the obligations or duties of the nurse in the nurse-patient relationship?

What's the most effective approach to get children to cooperate?

How public do you make known your personal ethics?

How do you deal with people outside? At a party you're beseiged by questions.

How do you deal with the other staff—differences and limits of responsibility?

How about physical contact? Can you literally be a shoulder to cry on, hold his hand if he's frightened?

As a student nurse, how do you exhibit confidence in front of a patient if you really don't have any?

Resentment felt by other hospital workers. Should a nurse make excuses for rotten colleagues to the patient?

After treating a patient for a while, how would you keep yourself emotionally uninvolved, so if a tragedy happened it wouldn't affect you?

How about the elderly patients that keep saying they want to die, but you know they're not going to for a while?

How may the nurse interact with foreign-speaking patients?

How friendly may the nurse become with the patient?

How much should you tell the patient, especially if he's asking the questions?

How do we deal with the different classes and personalities of patients?

How do you deal with patient's family; or do you leave that up to the doctor?

How do you deal with a patient that's going to die very soon and knows it?

Legally, what can a nurse do in an accident outside?

How do you deal with a young patient who's going to die and doesn't know it?

How much should a nurse take upon herself without doctor's orders? This includes psychological stimulation, etc.

How do you deal with death?

Different roles of the nurse.

How to deal with a patient who's a nurse or doctor?

What effect does the nurse-patient relationship have on physical prognosis?

Way of caring for "pain-in-the-neck" patient.

How do you go about terminating a relationship when you become attached to somebody?

What to do when the patient wants a lot of your time and you have other duties?

Do embarrassing situations (with male patients) continue to bother a nurse? Also, would any kind of illness affect the nurse?

How do you care for a patient who dosen't want to be cared for?

Medical persons' role in war, riot, social strife.

How do you cope with chronic complainers?

Treatment of people with knife and gunshot wounds.

What should the nurse do when she sees the doctor doing something wrong?

How to deal with fellow staff members on personal ethics (ignoring the patient, etc.).

How to deal with a patient addicted to narcotics who asks for more than he needs for pain.

What do you do when an instructor or head nurse insults you in front of patients?

This class of beginners in nursing, most of whom had never been in a hospital, covered in response to one question the gamut of vital areas in nurse-patient relations. Any teacher who makes the course responsive to these concerns will have a class of involved and interested students who *want* what they are getting in school. (Who is the teacher who does not dream of such classes?)

In the process of teaching to these responses, we dealt with the nature of the profession and the image of the individual nurse; endemic social stereotyping; the problem of face-to-face communication; institutional hierarchies and taboos; and the human need to reach out and touch. In other words, during the semester we encompassed the broadest professional problems (like treating moribund patients) and the most individually oriented solutions (like what to do when a patient makes a pass at you), not because I had a curriculum that I felt obliged to "cover," but because the students themselves were searching for answers to these problems.

Another time, with a group of experienced nurses, I asked the same question: "What do you want to know about nurse-patient relationships?" Their responses were often surprisingly similar, but just as often reflected the accumulated years of professional experience represented in the group:

Communication.

We need more skills in answering questions.

How much to tell the patient.

How to prevent misunderstanding on the part of the patient because of things he has overheard hospital personnel say.

What do you say to a patient who asks you if he's going to die?

How do you establish trusting relationships with children when doctors tell them things about their illness and you tell them something else because you don't know what the doctor has said?

What can you say when a doctor tells a patient something and the patient asks you if it's true, and you know it isn't true?

What do you say to a patient who says he wants to die?

What do you do when you don't understand the patient's language?

Just how much responsibility do you have to the patient's family? How far should you go in helping them adjust to the patient and his illness?

How do you deal with doctors who think all nurses are stupid?

How do you deal with prejudice?

What do you think of supervisors and doctors who bawl you out in front of patients?

Should professional people call each other by their first names when patients are present?

What about nurses who come right out of college and want to change everything?

Do you always have to keep your moral values to yourself?

How can you tell if you're prejudiced and don't know it?

I have difficulty hiding my feelings when I know a child is going to die.

How far do you go to change outdated practices?

What do you do about a patient who doesn't want you to care for him? How much do you insist?

I do less and less actual nursing. I'm not sure I like this.

In the course of exploring systematically each response and each concern, other interests became apparent and additional questions were raised in both groups. Thus, out of the response "Professionalism. What does it mean and what is the purpose of it?" came a discussion of how the concept of professionalism is used to discourage deviations from traditional practice. The nurse who suggests to the doctor that he is doing the patient a disservice by avoiding his questions is called "unprofessional"; the nurse who communicates to a patient her sorrow at his pain is "unprofessional." The term is used so arbitrarily and so obviously for the purpose of resisting change that many young people coming into nursing use the word with a sneer and imply that professionalism is an archaism that deserves no serious discussion. Others are re-defining professionalism in terms of knowledge, skill, and sensitivity and putting skills in human relations high on the list of the true professional.

Consistent with this view is the conclusion of one of my classes that honesty is a vital aspect of good human relations. So it becomes "professional" to express feelings about suffering, to answer direct questions put by patients, to protest the dishonesty of colleagues, and to resist the exploitation of one's self and of others in the name of "order," "tradition," or superior power. This single response to the problem census question became the basis for an intense consideration of a broad complex of values that undergird specific nursing practices. These values may well be the determining factors in the process of change in the profession. Coupled with skills in acting on these values, the whole nature of nurse-patient relation-ships may change radically.

For example, if the nurse maintains that she must be free to use her own judgment in answering patients' questions, and if she is willing to assume the responsibility for any errors in judgment, then she must engage in on-going consultation with the patient's physician so that both physician and nurse are in possession of the same information on which such judg-ments must be based. The nurse, then, becomes much more than a taker of orders. Nor does she find herself in the position of hedging or equivocating when questioned because she doesn't know what the doctor has told the patient.

One group of twenty graduate nurses who had been summoned by administrators to an in-service workshop in nurse-patient relations sat in their chairs and stared at me when I asked them what they wanted to know about nurse-patient relations. I don't know who suffered more, they or I, while I just stood there waiting for responses. I smiled first at one then at another. By my manner and my look of pleasant expectation I tried to communicate that I really did want to know the answers to the question, and that I was not at all disturbed at having to wait while they thought about it. But wait I would!

Finally, one of the nurses could stand it no longer and took a risk to break the silence:

How do you get your patients to cooperate?

I wrote the response on the chalk board and turned back to the group again. After a short wait, the questions continued:

How can you maintain control over your feelings when a child asks you if he's going to die—when you know he is?

How do you get an old person who doesn't want to live to take a hand in his own recovery?

What do you do when you know an L.P.N. is incompetent?

What do you do when you know an R.N. is incompetent?

What do you do when you know a doctor is incompetent? [Nervous laughs]

I've noticed that most people are very uncomfortable when they have to talk to a patient who is dying. How professional is *that?*

How do you help a young woman who thinks her life is over because she had a leg amputated?

I'm tired of being made to feel I don't know anything just because I'm new on the job.

Some people think they know everything just because they've read a book lately.

And that was the end of the problem census. I did not think it would be very difficult to plan experiences to help the group explore the problems they had so clearly identified. And I was right. We had a productive eight sessions, and when I finally left the group they were planning to make such sessions a regular part of their work schedule.

Recently, I conducted a problem census with part of the staff of a hospital. There were several interesting factors in this situation that, I think, are relevant to our concern with the education of nurses. One factor was that the group was made up of registered nurses, nurses' assistants, laboratory technicians, a pharmacist, a biophysicist, a psychiatrist, several people who did the cleaning, several who did minor repair work, an engineer, and several other job categories that I was not able to identify. This was quite a departure from the usual basis for selecting participants for an in-service workshop. Generally—in most professions—we limit the membership to people in the same or very similar professional category. I think the participants at this workshop were first surprised and then pleased at finding themselves together. I must confess to sharing their feelings. In addition, I learned something about the opportunities for productive communication in health care teams that has served me well in my work.

Another interesting factor was that the census was taken *after* I had worked with the group for three hours, providing some experiences that encouraged them to explore various aspects of race relations. I had never done a census at this particular point in my relationship with a group of people, but I had several reasons for such a procedure at this time: (1) Since there was no expectation that I would meet with the group again, I wanted to build some basis for continuity into that first meeting. By ending the session with a problem census, I was able to leave with the group a list of problems that they had said concerned them. If only one or two people felt that the list was justification enough for meeting again, they could assume the initiative for convening another session and the group could get to work on dealing with the problems. (2) From what I knew of the nature of such situations (a very large medical facility from which a diverse group was selected for a variety of reasons to participate in this seminar), I thought it was very unlikely that I would get many responses to such a question at the very beginning of the session. This was the first time these people had met; most of them had never spoken to one another as peers; their peer communication was hampered by the nature of our socio-economic system, which does not recognize the possibility of peer relationships between, for example, a biophysicist and a maintenance man.

I must also admit that I felt the need to provide a measure of safety for the people in the group, because I did not know just how secure they felt from reprisals by authority or resentment from one another. Also, since I was not going to continue working with them, I would have no opportunity to help them deal with any perilous consequences that might befall them as a result of the census. Therefore, I asked them to write their answers quickly, one to a card, and to drop their cards into a basin on the floor. (Subsequently, I had the responses typed in a list, duplicated, and distributed to them.) This is the list I distributed:

Responses to the Question: What Problems in Race Relations Are You Aware of in Your Working Situation?

0 (This is a rather ambiguous response; it may mean "There are no problems," or "I prefer not to identify any problems.")

Not being allowed to read bulletins or other information data because "I didn't think *you people*" would be interested.

How can we deemphasize size and color in supervising others or working with others?

Being black in any work situation or institution often creates problems of racism. Why should this be so?

Better understanding among people such as has resulted from this class.

Promotions are made on bases other than job qualifications and abilities.

White volunteers catering to only white patients.

"You people think you can get away with everything." (White woman to black man.)

Jewish supervisor actually told me he would sooner promote another Jew because "they have been discriminated against so much in the past."

The fiscal department doesn't have any black employees.

The credit union had a meeting. The question came up why no black people were on the board. One lady officer said, "This is the way it is and we're not changing."

Black employees "making fun" of *only* white employees.

White head supervisor always picks the only white supervisor to attend classes or meetings with him, eliminating other supervisors who are black.

Injured on the job and had to take my sick leave days and was criticized for taking sick leave. And explained I looked too healthy to believe I was really hurt.

Barrier to communication created by defensiveness of members of both races—creating decision-making schism on basis of race rather than personal philosophy.

Upgrade more black employees in the Engineering Department at this hospital.

Supervisors should come to these workshops.

Executive order emphasizes promotions of the Blacks. This is prejudice in reverse and has aroused consternation.

Have more interracial interaction meetings such as this one.

Attitudes on the job. Situations involving Black men and White women, and vice versa.

Telling ethnic jokes on the worksite.

Remarks from superiors such as, "I don't know what more they want."

Older employee tries to indoctrinate newer workers to her anti-black bias within the office.

It seems that the black people in this place get the dirty jobs.

Get the white guy to do it this time.

It becomes clear from experience with the problem census technique that there is really no need for an instructor or group leader to assume the whole responsibility for developing a course in nurse-patient relations. Given an opportunity, the students as well as the experienced nurses will express a wide range of concerns, study of which will provide them with knowledge, skills, and sensitivities that the effective nurse needs on the job.

OTHER TECHNIQUES
FOR ENCOURAGING PARTICIPATION

The non-evaluative, accepting atmosphere generated by the problem census is a good one in which to practice other participatory skills. Participation in the educational setting involves raising questions, answering questions, gathering data, and solving problems. What can the teacher or group leader do—or not do—to encourage such participation by students or group members? The problem census technique embodies the necessary behaviors: using students' responses, dealing with attacking criticism, and asking questions and waiting for the answers.

Using Students' Responses

Just as the problem census requires making a record of students' responses and using those responses as the "curriculum" for the course, so there are other methods that are equally effective in helping students take an active part in their own education. One thing that both instructors and fellow students can practice is taking a person's response and building on it, enlarging on it, adding a new dimension to it, pairing it with another idea or another experience. What we too often do with other people's remarks is

(1) merely wait until they are finished so we can say what *we* have to say;
(2) interrupt them so that the complete idea is never heard. Those people
who are not very aggressive in group discussion, we just never give a chance
to speak at all. Consequently, many group discussions become meaningless
exercises that produce no more than a collection of individual observations
that would be held even if the people never got together to "discuss."

The value of the group discussion lies in the opportunity it provides
for educational and creative experience not available in the same way to
someone who is working alone. The product of the group—whether it is the
solution of a situational problem or a plan of operation of some kind—
must be more than the sum of the contributions of the individual group
members. A response by one person may trigger an idea from another
that he might never have thought of alone; the organizing skill of one person
may integrate the discrete contributions of four others into a new and
exciting approach to the problem at hand.

However, people are not born with the building skills necessary
for working in groups productively; one way or another they need to learn
those skills. Here is an exercise that may help them.

An instructor can start with a class of twenty-five or thirty to
demonstrate the exercise, and then break up the class into groups of nine
or ten to continue practicing in a more realistic setting for problem solving.
Pick a topic; one item from the problem census would be suitable. (It is
advisable to pick a subject that most people have opinions about and voice
rather easily. It is best to avoid extremely emotional subjects for use in skill
practice sessions because the combination of an emotionally charged topic
and the frustration felt in learning a new skill are often too much to deal
with at once.) Say to the class:

> "Let us discuss for ten minutes the topic from your problem
> census: *How can we deal with sexism?* While you discuss, I will be
> looking to see if some of you have a certain discussion skill. Everytime
> someone demonstrates that skill, I will identify that person. At the
> end of five minutes, we'll see if you know what skill I'm looking for.
> Remember, the skill has nothing to do with the knowledge of the
> subject of sexism; it has to do only with the ability to discuss."

The class begins its discussion. After a minute or two, during which
half a dozen random remarks are made by the students, one of them says,
"You know, Jane, I'm surprised you feel that way about it, too. I've been
thinking that I'm the only one who ever had such an experience."

The instructor says, "Ann Collins has the skill I'm looking for."
She says nothing more. After a few self-conscious giggles, the discussion
continues.

A few minutes later, Jim Brown offers an observation: "If a woman feels good about herself, is proud of being what she is, then no sexist attitudes can bother her too much."

Elaine responds: "I agree with you, Jim. A person needs a positive self-concept if she is to live up to her potential in our kind of society. But don't you think that, even with a good opinion of herself, she can still be deprived of equal opportunities by prejudice and discrimination?" The instructor says: "Elaine Black has the skill I'm looking for." The discussion continues.

If no one demonstrates the skill, the instructor may use the examples here to illustrate what he is looking for and then continue with the exercise in the same way.

After the ten minutes are up, the instructor says, "Let us stop here for a few minutes. You will be able to go on with your discussion in a little while. Now, what is the discussion skill I've been looking for?"

Student #1:	Listening to what other people say.
Instructor:	That's part of it.
Student #2:	Agreeing with another person.
Instructor:	That's part of the skill, too.
Student #3:	What's so great about agreeing with everybody?
Student #2:	It makes you feel good when people aren't always cutting you down.
Student #3:	You don't have to cut someone down, but you don't have to always agree either. You never get anywhere just by agreeing. What if you honestly have a completely different point of view?
Student #2:	I didn't say *always* agree.
Student #4:	It's important to state another point of view, and you're right, you can do it without destroying the person you disagree with. But if it's possible you can see what there is in what someone else says that sort of relates to what you have to say.
Student #5:	Yeah, like receiving the ball and running with it!
Student #1:	We just demonstrated it again!
Instructor:	All right, that's the idea. Now let's practice it. We'll continue the discussion for twenty minutes, but this time no one can say anything unless he can find something in what the previous speaker has said and relate it to what he has to say. We'll break up into small groups so that everyone will have a better chance to participate. (The instructor should sit in with one of the groups and participate in the skill practice, too.)

At the end of the session, the class might consider what their discussion group accomplished that they might not have if each member had merely been writing a composition on "How can we deal with sexism?" As with any practicing of skills, it is good to bear in mind that such opportunities must be provided regularly until the skill is learned and integrated into the person's normal behavior.

Dealing with Attack

One of the most pervasive reasons for students' reluctance to participate in class is the fear of being attacked by their peers or by the instructor. The building skills, that imply also listening and agreeing, help to reduce the incidence of attack. There are still, however, the problems of presenting opposing points of view and giving an individual feedback on his behavior in non-threatening ways, and of making an attacker aware of the effect of his behavior. To say to a person who constantly interrupts others and tends to "hold the floor" for long periods of time, "You've got a big mouth!" is, to say the least, not helpful. It is a destructive attack that encourages defensive behavior or a counter-attack. The person attacked can learn to say to such an attacker, "What you said makes me feel so bad I just want to run away from the group." Or someone not immediately involved can suggest, "Saying that really doesn't help her, it just insults her."

To present an opposing point of view as information and an expression of personal feeling is generally less threatening than trying to change the other person's point of view. To say, "I feel that . . ." or "I read that . . ." is more likely to be accepted by the other group members than, "You're wrong!" or "You don't know what you're talking about!" or "You shouldn't feel that way!"

The question is: How can we help people become aware of and practice the more open and trusting responses, and so encourage more participation in class? A part of one session might be devoted to collecting all the things people say in the course of discussion that hurt or anger other people. One way to do this and still preserve the safety and anonymity that a new group might need is to have students write down the remarks. Rather than trying to recall some remote discussion, the instructor divides the class up into groups of eight or nine people and asks them to solve a particular problem. At the end of the discussion, they are each given a pack of small papers or cards and asked to write—one to a card—all the things that were said and done that they thought were attacking and destructive. As each card is completed, it is tossed into a receptacle in the middle of the room.

The cards are then redistributed to the groups. In each group, one card at a time is turned up, read aloud, and discussed in an attempt to understand why the remark or behavior on it was felt to be aggressive.

Then the group tries to find alternative ways of responding in specific situations without attacking.

The next time that each group is posed a problem for discussion, they are asked to keep in mind the attacking responses and the alternatives they found. Each time somebody feels attacked, or thinks someone has attacked, he may give some pre-arranged sign, like pitching a penny into the center of the circle, or sticking a thumbtack into a corkboard on the floor in the center of the circle. Then the person who has made the attacking remark must backtrack and use one of the alternatives. If he cannot think of an alternative, the group may help him.

Here is an interesting problem that may be used for the discussion in this exercise:

The Dialysis Machines

You nine people make up the total professional staff of a small isolated hospital. Because there is no doctor closer than 200 miles, all of you have been trained to deliver primary health care. You have contact with a doctor by short-wave radio, but you haven't seen him for eight months.

In your community at this time there are seven people suffering from a variety of kidney diseases. None of them is able to move to the city for long-term treatment. Suddenly, it becomes clear that four of these people need immediate continuous dialysis if they are to survive. A fifth one—a physician who had been vacationing in the mountains nearby when he was hurt in an accident—also needs the machine. The hospitals has two small machines, and there is no hope of obtaining any more in the near future.

Since only two patients can be treated, the three untreated ones will die. In twenty-five minutes, decide which two people of the five will be put on dialysis:

1. A wife, six months pregnant
2. A fifty-year-old Catholic priest
3. A Black man, husband, father of four small children
4. A famous musician
5. The vacationing doctor

It is, of course, not necessary to use the same problem for the whole class in order to isolate the attacking responses. In the process of exploring their different interests, each group inevitably engages in discussion. At one point, the instructor may merely intercede and ask the students to participate in the exercise, using the responses in their most recent discussion as the source of their data.

Setting the Scene

Sometimes students need to be convinced that the institution—
and the instructor—really mean it when they say that they want active
student participation in planning and pursuing the course of study. It is not
so easy to convince them when they are ushered into a classroom where the
seats are neatly arranged in rows all facing a chalkboard or a stage
and the instructor is positioned in front of the room in the traditional
information-disseminating stance. No matter what announcement the
instructor makes about "This is *your* course; I want you to feel free to
decide how the course will be conducted," what he is really announcing by
the furniture arrangement is, "You will speak only to me," and "I am
standing up at the front of the room because I am the leader of this group
and the authority is vested in me."

I handle the matter in two ways: (1) I absolutely refuse to conduct
any class in a room that has seats bolted to the floor; I have, consequently,
met my classes in some very odd places, like a boiler room and a clinical-
practice room that had three or four beds in it. (2) I come to the room ten
or fifteen minutes early each day and pile all the chairs against the walls
so that we may use the cleared space in the center. (Once I drew the
curtains on the stage and used the *stage* for the class—a lovely, cosy setting
that had passers-by wondering what was going on back there!)

How the students arrange themselve each day must depend on the
nature of the activities they are engaged in. Should there be fifty students
in the class, you might want to ask them to break up into small groups in
order to decide which items in the problem census they want to work on.
In this activity, some groups may sit on the floor (if there is a carpet on
the floor!); others may pull chairs away from the wall and arrange
them in circles. Still others may want to go into the corridor or an adjacent
room because they prefer a lower noise level. Since in such cases the
instructor must be available to raise questions (Don't those items you've
selected represent a very broad range of subjects? Can you do them all
justice?), offer alternatives (If your interests are so different from the others,
perhaps you'd like to work with another group?), act as resource person
(There's a very good film on that in the public library), and in other ways
to facilitate the work of the students, she cannot maintain a fixed position
at the head of the class. She must circulate from group to group, sitting
in and participating in one group, while being ready to respond to calls for
help from the others.

I remember the startled look on the face of a colleague who
passed by the open door of my room one day and saw the students sitting
and lying around the room, on chairs, prone on the floor with their heads
together, or cross-legged on the stage. The fact that two of those sitting on

the floor wore nun's habits did not help to reduce the startled response, but she did have to admit that everyone seemed to be very much absorbed in what was going on in his group.

Even I must laugh at the memory of one class that met in the room with beds. After we had role-played a problem situation and were discussing the consequences of various proposed solutions, I suddenly became aware of the physical arrangements: One student was lying on the bed, just as the role-playing had left her; another was sitting cross-legged at her feet; a third sat on another bed, feet dangling; several were ranged along the top of a wheeled cart that threatened to take off every time one of them made an emphatic statement. But they were *involved!* They were really struggling with this problem, and the absence of physical constriction seemed to free them to immerse themselves totally in the professional problem before them.

Providing Alternative Activities

It is not difficult to get a small number of people in any group to participate actively. Always there are individuals who cannot submit passively to any imposition of system or authority. However, an instructor who is searching for ways to involve all of her students might consider some student needs and their implications for learning.

1. *It is not reasonable to expect every student to be interested in the same topic at the same time.*

If the instructor can accept this as true, then he will provide opportunities for students to work in areas that they are interested in at a particular time. This does not mean that they will never learn about other things that are needed to do the professional job; it just means that they will come to those other things at different times and in different ways.

Let us take, for example, the responses on the first problem census in this chapter. Suppose twenty students would like to find answers to questions about the nursing care of children; twelve students are concerned with relationships with administrators, supervisors, and other nurses; and eight students want to learn how to deal with patients' stereotypic perceptions of nurses. One student wants to explore attitudes about death. Nine students seem unable to make a decision, and seem to want to gather around the instructor and be told what is important for them.

While the other students begin to explore in small groups just how they want to proceed, those students around the instructor are reassured that, before the end of the term, they will "cover" every subject area that they will need to function on the job. They are then urged to pick one census item that seems important to them. Some move off to find the appropriate groups; others decide to work alone.

The instructor unobtrusively goes to one group and listens while they justify their interest in studying attitudes about death. Each one tells of a personal experience—an ignored patient, an evasive physician, a family unable to cope. They are on their way: they are trying to define the nature of their concern, and a meaningful way to start is by talking about personal experiences and remembered feelings. The teacher moves off to another group.

Here a feeling of frustration has already begun to build. One person wants to develop a list of nursing functions so that "patients will know what a nurse is supposed to be and not expect her to be something else." Another person is rejecting this idea as "ridiculous" and asks, "What good is a list? Who's going to read it besides us?" Another person feels they should "do some reading on the subject." Still another keeps insisting that nurses stereotype patients! The teacher pulls up a chair and listens quietly for a few minutes. How can she help them make a decision about first steps in the process?

"Perhaps," the teacher finally suggests, "what you have here are several sub-topics. Perhaps you ought to divide the work up and then come back together to share what you have."

"I'd like to do a little reading on this," says one student. And then, turning to the teacher, "Do you know of any books or articles?"

"Yes, I have several titles I can let you have. Each one will suggest others to you. Come to my office when you're ready."

"I'm ready now," she says, poised to escape from the frustration in the group.

"Don't you want to know what the other people in your group will be doing?"

She shrugs her shoulders and then responds to the urging of a friend in the group, "Let's all decide what we're going to do and then set a time for getting together again."

The teacher smiles with satisfaction and moves away, only to be stopped by a student sitting alone. And so it goes until the session is over for the day. But the interest and the involvement does not end with the bell. As a matter of fact, the teacher leaves while the students are still making their final arrangements with one another.

The instructor need not be concerned if she is able to work with only one or two groups during this session. She must keep reminding herself that her students have had many years experience in studying: they know a great deal about gathering information. She should also bear in mind that they are working on topics they are interested in; even if their research skills are mediocre, their interest will keep them going at least until she has the time to give them specific assistance. Above all, it is useful to hold to the truism that there is very little "instant learning" in the classroom. The efficiently written and delivered lecture may cover the whole subject but it does not ensure that the whole subject will be learned. Struggling with the learning process, the students are involved in a dynamic learning experience that will have meaning for them long after their lecture notes have faded.

2. *Students have different learning styles, and what may be effective teaching for one student will be a waste of time for another student.*

If a student is firmly convinced that the only way to learn a subject is to read the authorities on that subject, he will not lend himself immediately to that phase of the educational process that relies on students' sharing their feelings. To him this approach may be a waste of time, perhaps partly because he is reluctant to make this kind of contribution. However, if he can start by arming himself with some "facts" from books, he can become a part of the group initially by sharing what he has read. As he becomes more comfortable, he may begin to see the value of other kinds of "facts"—like "feelings."

On the other hand, a student who feels that the books are "irrelevant" may become aware eventually that writers of books are also people who have had experiences and who have feelings—people whose lifetimes may be added to our own to give us the benefit of more than one person's perceptions.

3. *Students probably learn more from one another than they do from their instructors.*

As students gather information and share it with others—express feelings, tell about experiences, interview authorities, and read books—each one becomes not only a learner but also a teacher of the others. Because it is often easier to argue with peers, challenge their points of view, and offer one's own point of view, the teaching-learning process is a much more dynamic one than the traditional interaction is between student and teacher, with the communication arrows generally pointing from teacher to student.

The teacher need have no fear that the students will overlook his value as a resource person in the course. They know his background, they are aware that he has special skills and knowledge; and as their own sophistication in the subject grows, they will probably be asking the "expert" more and more significant questions.

Asking Questions

One of the ways in which teachers reduce participation in the learning process is by asking questions and not giving students time to answer them. One of the ways in which students discourage participation is by neglecting to ask one another questions. Let me explain this point further.

In conducting the problem census, one of the hard-and-fast rules

is that the *exact* wording of the question must not be changed. The tendency
of many teachers is to ask a question, wait a second or so, and then re-word
the question—or even change it completely. Those students who are very
quick to answer manage to get an answer in before the change, and another
answer after each change. Most of the students, however, need a little more
time—to think, to muster courage, to arrange their words—and they are
the ones who rarely get a chance to answer. Generally, we label them
"non-participants," without being aware that we are setting them up for
non-participation.

   We see this kind of teacher behavior reflected in student/student
behavior. When students do ask one another questions, the questions are
largely rhetorical. At any rate, the questioner rarely gives anyone time
to answer before he is off and talking again.

   One way of dealing with this problem is to have people actually
practice asking questions and waiting for the answers—and then using
those answers. The students arrange themselves in groups of eight or nine
to discuss a topic, perhaps one of the items from the problem census. They
may proceed with the discussion in the usual way, except that a person may
not speak until he has first asked a question of someone else in the group
and has received his answer. The answer must then be used in some way by
the questioner: added to, built upon, challenged, and so on. At first, people
may ask any question just so that they may get the chance to say what they
want to say. However, as they begin to realize that such a procedure is
exploitative and unfair to the person questioned, the questions become more
meaningful. (The realization that they are using people unfairly comes
largely from their own feelings when this is done to them.)

Developing Trust

   The activities designed to provide practice in participation also
raise the level of trust in a group. If we reduce attack, accept and use
students' contributions, ask questions that we really want answered, and
provide for individual interests and learning styles, we are, in effect, saying
that we care, we appreciate, and we really want to know one another.
It is on such behaviors that we build our trust. When we are with people
who see us as having feelings and responding to needs, we feel less risk in
establishing relationships; and what small risk we do feel, we are willing
to take.

   There are other classroom behaviors that also tend to reduce risk
in interacting and that can be systematically practiced until they become a
part of us.

   1. The instructor must resist the constant compulsion to evaluate

every student response. And students must likewise resist evaluating everything the instructor says. Everyone in the classroom must live free of the
expectation that everything he says will be labeled "good" or "bad," rather
than just heard and responded to. Those who are, for one reason or another,
reluctant to risk such evaluation certainly do not contribute to the group
everything they are capable of contributing. They simply do not trust the
others enough to risk offering a contribution for fear it will be rejected.

Perhaps this lack of trust underlies the reluctance of most teachers
to lower the barriers between themselves and their students. Perhaps if they
could trust students not to pounce on their errors or take advantage of their
friendliness they might more readily abandon the podium and the chalkboard and sit down side by side with their students.

One exercise for helping develop such trust might be to ask two
or three people in the class to act as observers during a whole session and
count the number of times people evaluated one another instead of using
one another's contributions. The awareness that observers are counting
helps people reduce the tendency to evaluate. Within a short time, a person
who evaluates, or one who is evaluated, is likely to announce to the class:
"There I go again!" or "You're evaluating me!"

2. The instructor must stop playing the teacher game. And, again,
the students must stop playing the student game. What I call "the teacher
game" is the mystique that many teachers feel they must maintain if they
are to be effective in the classroom. This involves keeping a certain distance
between themselves and students; repressing all display of spontaneous
emotion, like a burst of anger; sharing information about students with other
faculty members while keeping such information from the student; never
admitting that they might not know something; never confessing to having
feelings of doubt or fear. In short, teachers are usually interested in presenting to students a one-dimensional façade that is consistent with the
stereotype of the teacher. This pose is often called being "professional" and
has its counterpart in some of the definitions of "professional" that nurses
use. To me, it seems to be "un-human," to coin a term.

Faced with this kind of pretense, students engage in a game of their
own: work only for grades, get away with as much as you can, find chinks
in the teacher's armor, and pretend that you're serious about school when
you know very well that school has little to do with real life.

Given the kinds of open cooperative behaviors discussed in this
chapter, students and teachers may reach the point of trust and mutual
respect wherein such games will be unnecessary.

2 *THE IDEAL NURSE,*
THE IDEAL PATIENT,
AND OTHER STEREOTYPES

WHAT NURSES EXPECT

Although games are fun, there is no reason why they cannot be used to facilitate learning. As a matter of fact, a little fun in the learning situation helps to ease the tension generated by exploring unfamiliar territory and experimenting with new behaviors. Instructors may protest that learning is a serious business—especially learning a profession in which practices can have life-and-death consequences. But serious need not be equated with grim. At any rate, the informality and the give and take of a game situation encourage the timid to participate, provide an opportunity for the more active to assume leadership, and betray the cynical into giving a little of themselves.

Here is a game that helps to bring out into the open student expectations about nursing. People come into the profession with the beliefs and feelings that are held in the general society. Much of the anxiety generated in new students is caused by the dawning realization that what they expect a nurse to be is unrealistic. Many students have great difficulty reconciling their idea of what a nurse should be and their disappointment that they can never measure up to that ideal. Interestingly enough, their expectation of what makes an ideal patient seems to persist throughout their careers, with attendant deleterious effects on their relationships with patients and the quality of nursing care they provide. The pervasive use of such terms as "crock" and "temperamental" and "uncooperative" give a clue to what nurses look for in their patients. Here, too, there is apparent conflict between the intellectual formulations in the profession and the personal-emotional responses of individual nurses. Like the teaching profession that claims to teach "the whole child," the nursing profession "recognizes" that a patient does not abandon his personality at the door of the hospital. It maintains that the sick person must be brought to independence as soon as possible—that independence is an important factor in his convalescence. Its teachers lecture in classes that the needs of the individual patient must not be totally subordinate to the necessity for hospital "efficiency."

However, as in education, so in nursing the gap between what we know and what we do is wide indeed. The often discouraging point is reached when we hear practitioners rationalizing away the gap, offering all kinds of "good reasons" why it is necessary to keep doing what we know is not desirable for the child—or for the patient. I think it is preferable, when we do not put our own knowledge into practice, to admit that we are unable to do so for one reason or another, rather than to maintain stoutly that to put that knowledge to use is not practical. In the first instance, we are left free to search for ways to translate our knowledge into practice; in the second, we abandon all hope of change.

Part of the picture of the nurse in our society involves misconceptions concerning morality and sexuality. Such misconceptions, although rejected intellectually by student nurses, are yet maintained on an emotional level and cause inner conflict and anxiety about assuming the identity of nurse. It is not easy for the woman nurse to maintain her professional poise when she is faced with a patient who assumes she is "fast," unfeeling, tough, and wise in ways that diminish her right to respect.

Paradoxically, yet side by side with these misconceptions, is the prevalent expectation that nurses are completely selfless, self-sacrificing, totally devoted to their patients to the exclusion of their private lives and personal concerns. Nurses often encounter this attitude when they seek higher salaries or try to improve undesirable working conditions. It comes almost as a shock to some people that nurses should so far forget their commitment to humanity as to demand a reasonable standard of living!

The game:

1. Every member of the class is given a packet of twenty-five or thirty small cards or pieces of paper.

2. The instructor or a class member poses the question, "What are the qualities of the ideal patient?"

The class is first asked to name *categories* of qualities and the instructor writes these categories on the board. Examples of such categories are *beliefs, feelings, personality, race, religion, nationality, "interests," skills, appearance, behaviors, attitudes, philosophy of life,* and so on.

The instructor writes these categories on the chalkboard.

3. The class takes fifteen minutes to write down, *one to a paper,* all the qualities of the ideal patient that they can think of, covering as many of the listed categories as possible.

At the end of the fifteen-minute period, the papers are collected and put aside.

4. The class then takes fifteen minutes to write down, *again one to a paper,* all the qualities of the ideal nurse. Then these papers are collected.

5. The class divides into two teams that line up facing each other. (They should, of course, be comfortably seated, since this is essentially a discussion game. In the past, especially with large classes, some of the people have sat in chairs, others on the floor in front of the chairs, to ensure maximum face-to-face positioning as well as an air of informality that encouraged people to turn and look at one another frequently, to speak without waiting for permission, and to forget the subduing effect of the classroom.)

6. The cards containing the patient traits are distributed to one team. The other team gets the cards listing the nurse traits. Each person, then, has a small stack of traits to play with.

7. The instructor, or perhaps a class member who has had some patient-care experience, acts as moderator and judge.

8. One person on the first team reads an ideal patient trait from a card.

Any person on the other team who has a card with a nurse trait that is "good" for that patient calls it out. Then he must justify why the nurse with the trait is ideal for that patient.

Members of the first team must try to find errors in attempted justification, proving in their turn that the nurse trait is *not* suitable for such a patient.

9. The judge calls time to end the argument (never longer than three or four minutes) and decides which team has won the point.

At the end of the session, the team with the most points wins. Then the class might profitably spend some time sharing what they have learned from playing the game. In these post-game discussions in the past, students have had some interesting reactions. One once observed, "It's silly to expect any one person to have all the perfect qualities. Nurses are only human, and so are patients." Another speculated that it might be worthwhile to consider individual traits when assigning nurses to patients. In this way an irritable patient might be better served by a mild, easy-going nurse; and the nurse with the short fuse might work better with a relatively calm, undemanding patient. (Obviously it would not be possible to arrange perfect matches all the time, but some attempt could be made to reduce the possibility of putting together people who are bound to have difficulty in interacting harmoniously. Here is one way in which human needs are given preferential consideration over "efficient" management.)

One student surprised herself when she put into words all the traits that she expected nurses to have—and, by implication, that she expected herself to have. She had never realized before that the ideal she held was unattainable and that if she persisted in maintaining it she was doomed to failure. She confessed that she had had, as a child, a beloved grandmother who was tended by a nurse until she died. The family had talked often about "that angel" who had cared so selflessly for the old woman, and seemed to imply to the immature perceptions of the child that the angel never ate or slept or engaged in other worldly pursuits while her patient lingered.

Some of the qualities nursing students seem to expect of nurses, and of themselves, do approach the angel level! The student who wrote that her picture of the ideal nurse was one who liked herself, loved people, was poised, happy, cooperative, never nasty, enthusiastic, optimistic, dedicated, stable, consistent, soft-spoken but firm, and with an out-going personality, really believed with the poet that "a man's reach should exceed his grasp . . .!" But when she added that the ideal nurse is *white,* she introduced a factor that gives us a clue to the genesis of all such expectations.

THE NURSE AS A STEREOTYPE: WHAT PATIENTS EXPECT

Just as nurses have absorbed the stereotype of the nurse from the attitudes and expectations of our society, so the patients have absorbed the same stereotype in the same way. One white woman recently admitted to the hospital, and experiencing some discomfort, rang for a nurse. The new shift had just come on, and one of the nurses came in, smiling, to help. The woman's response was, "I don't want you. Send me a real nurse!" Not only did she think that all RNs were white, but she assumed that a Black woman in uniform must be a practical nurse or an aide!

Despite the advantages men seem to enjoy within the profession, they must still deal with the problems created by a society that sees nurses only as women. The woman patient who refuses care from a male nurse, the male patient who questions the sexuality of the male nurse, families and friends who raise their eyebrows and look skeptical or incredulous when a man announces his intention of becoming a nurse—all these people reflect the widespread belief that nurses should be women and that any deviation from this expectation is somehow abnormal.

Curiously enough, the angel of mercy stereotype of the nurse is held by some patients simultaneously with a quite different attitude. Feeling helpless in the hospital and at the mercy of hospital personnel for needed care, patients are often fearful of antagonizing nurses by making demands, asking for too much, or complaining about anything. They are afraid that when they desperately need help, the nurse will not come in answer to their ring because of pique or annoyance with the patients' behavior.

Nor are these the only views of nurses held by patients. The idea that nurses are hard and tough and insensitive to suffering seems to conflict with the caring, sensitive, dedicated image of the nurse that is also part of the stereotype. But this is the curious nature of human thinking: we do not seem overly disturbed at holding to apparently opposite views at the same time. We manage merely to take out the view we need at any moment to bolster an observation or win an argument. When we want the other view for a similar purpose, it is ready in the appropriate compartment of the brain.

Of course, the idea that the female nurse (the stereotype has not yet included the male nurse in the same way) is fair game sexually for anyone who wants to make a pass at her is pretty widely held. One would think that a society that is so rapidly throwing off the shackles of Victorian prudery would also see through the misconception that knowledge of the human body and commitment to tending people physically causes essential changes in an individual's moral outlook. But no—the same people raised to admire Florence Nightingale also hold to such conclusions about any woman who becomes a nurse.

PROBLEMS OF RACE

Being reared in our kind of society predisposes us to see certain groups of people as restricted to certain niches in life. Whites, for example, have long accepted as "natural" the fact that Black people generally do not become doctors, lawyers, nurses, and other status professionals. (Those who do are, of course, the rare exceptions!) Intellectually, they may firmly endorse the American Creed that maintains that all men are equal. Emotionally, however, they find themselves accepting the policy of exclusion and are quite disturbed when it is breeched. If you are white and you would like to check out your own propensity toward this kind of attitude, imagine yourself being treated by a Black dentist. Honestly, now, would you consider having a Black dentist for yourself and your family? The chances are that your response falls somewhere between "It just never occurred to me to consider it" to "Black dentists are not as capable as white dentists." The response is, I think, predictable. Given a choice between a white and a Black dentist, you would pick the white one. It is on the level of feeling and the concomitant behavior that our belief in equality breaks down.

Consider the capable Black nurse in one hospital who worked in an apparently harmonious situation. She had just been promoted to supervisor and was pointed to with pride by administrators and nurses alike as evidence of the absence of discrimination in their hospital. She shook her head sadly when I asked her if everything was as good as I had been told it was. She had experienced considerable antagonism and resentment from her first day on the job. And she had even overheard a group of nurses attributing her promotion to the fact that she was Black.

I have talked to administrators who bemoaned the fact that so few Black students were applying for admission to nursing programs. They wanted so much to have "integrated" classes and were really rather fearful of being accused of excluding Black applicants because the classes were so overwhelmingly white. It seems to be true that disproportionately few Black women are applying for nursing programs. Part of the reason may lie in the past experience of Black applicants. A policy of systematic discrimination has blocked their way, and it takes time to make people aware of a change in policy and to convince them that their applications will get fair consideration.

It is also undoubtedly true that there still exists quotas for the admission of Blacks. That is, a hospital school or college decides that it must present an image of open acceptance and non-discrimination to the public. So they make a point of admitting one or two Black applicants. Usually, those admitted have been screened on the basis of criteria far more stringent than the other applicants are subjected to, so that the Black students admitted take on the aura of super-students who could not possibly be "unacceptable" to whites. Knowing that this sort of thing goes on discourages many Black people from considering nursing as a career.

Again, at this time in our history, many opportunities in business, industry, and the professions are opening up to Black people. With wider choice, young people are, quite frankly, choosing more lucrative jobs and more prestigious professions than nursing. Especially those who are really of superior ability and with special talents do not feel that they must become special recipients of nursing dispensations when other opportunities are open to them.

To balance the record, there are programs that are making special efforts to recruit and admit Black nursing applicants, and the efforts are paying off. Not only are Black students doing as well as white students have always done, but the presence of Black students has provided more useful opportunities for dealing with problems of interracial relations in nursing. This does not mean that an all-white group cannot concern itself with problems of race. It can, of course, develop insights and gather new information that can make future interracial contacts more satisfying and productive.

However, when there are both Black and white students in a class, then the opportunity—the first for many people—to exchange experiences and share feelings is presented. And there is no substitute for first-hand experience with members of other groups if we are to begin to solve the problems we have in interacting with one another.

We must be careful, however, that the few Black students in class are not made to bear the whole burden of the learning situation. It is not unusual for white students in a group to turn to the single Black student and ask, "How do Black people feel about . . .?" As if one person can presume to speak for all Black people!

Most Black people have learned to shrug off the question as merely additional evidence that whites think that all Blacks think alike. They often refuse to participate in the re-education of whites, maintaining that they are tired of the process, that misconception and prejudice is a white problem, and it is up to the whites to get their own heads together.

Some Black people, when faced with the white expectation that they speak for all Black people, simply set the record straight before they say what they have to say: "I can't speak for all Black people; I can speak only for myself. There are individuals who agree with me and others who disagree with what I believe." If the white students are really listening, they must quickly readjust their expectations and begin to question the idea of a "homogeneous" Black population.

Where Do You Stand?

It is not difficult for most of us to read, and agree with, the broad observations that condemn racism and advocate equality. However, how often do we really come face to face with our own attitudes? How receptive are we to evidence that we see people through a distorting haze of error and animosity? Here is a small experiment that you can conduct to gather such evidence.

Look at the hospital scene below. *Before you read beyond this paragraph,* write a brief description of what is happening in the picture.

Now that you have finished your description, complete the following checklist:

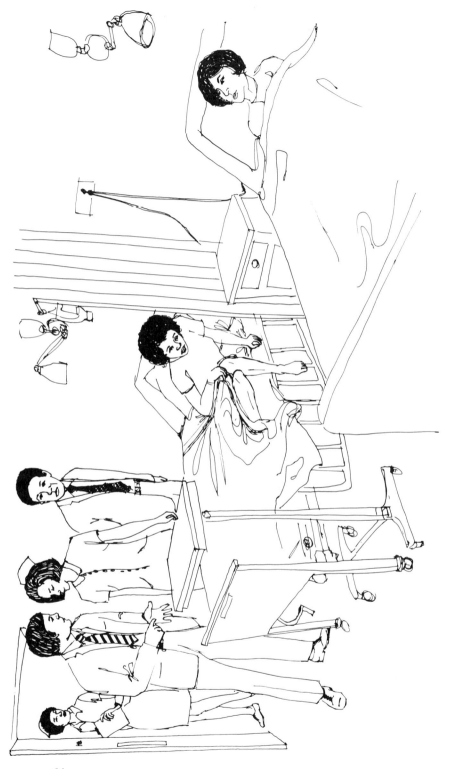

Perception Checklist

	Yes	No
1. Did you mention that there were both Black and white people in the scene?		
2. Did you say or imply that the white patient was upset in any way?		
3. Did you say or imply that the Black patient was upset in any way?		
4. Did you say or imply that the white patient was threatening, angry, or hostile?		
5. Did you say or imply that the Black patient was threatening, angry, or hostile?		
6. Did you say or imply that the white man standing was angry, threatening or hostile?		
7. Did you say that the white man was a doctor?		
8. Did you say or imply that the Black man standing was angry, threatening, or hostile?		
9. Did you say that the Black man was a doctor?		
10. Did you say or imply that the Black nurse at the door was angry, threatening, or hostile?		

If you never "noticed" that the people in the scene were of different races, you may stoutly argue that "race doesn't mean a thing to me. I treat everyone the same!" I am afraid that, as lofty a sentiment as this seems to be, it is analogous to maintaining that Americans live by the American Creed of equality. The evidence simply does not bear this out! Maybe there are some Americans who never notice another person's race; but of the hundreds of people who have said this to me, every single one eventually demonstrated clearly that the statement was not an accurate description of himself: (1) They confessed fear of Black people in certain situations but no fear of white people in exactly the same situations. (2) They believed things about all Black people that are not true about all Black people. (3) They ascribed different causative factors for the same behaviors, depending on whether the person was Black or white (for example, criminal behavior).

It is time that we realized that when we deny that race is significant to us we are not demonstrating our freedom from prejudice. In a society like ours, the people who do not notice race are not tolerant—they are unconscious! The denial usually indicates a lack of awareness of one's own behavior, for an observer can see very clearly that the person who does not notice race usually gives himself away.

If you answered yes to item 2 and no to item 3, you might ask yourself why. If you will look at the illustration again you will see that the expressions on the faces of both patients is very similar. As a matter of fact, the position of the Black patient might, at first glance, actually seem to indicate some agitation, whereas the white patient seems quiet and at rest. Did you, perhaps, displace your own feelings onto the white patient? Would *you*, perhaps, feel upset at the prospect of living in the same room with a Black person?

Did you answer yes to items 5, 8, and 10 and no to items 4 and 6? If you did, how does it happen that you see the Black people in the scene as threatening and hostile and the white people as not? It cannot be the expressions on the faces or the gestures because they are similar in both Blacks and whites. Do you, perhaps, feel frightened of Black people generally?

Conversely, if you answered no to items 5, 8, and 10 and yes to items 4 and 6, you might ask yourself if you see white people as generally threatening and hostile, even when there is no evidence of their hostility.

Did you answer yes to item 7 and no to item 9? Why? Does it seem more natural to have a white doctor than a Black doctor? So natural that you never even thought about it? (Did you ever consider that this kind of subtle expectation may operate in people who pass on medical school applications?) Or did you answer this way because you know very well that white men have a better chance of becoming doctors than Black men do?

Obviously, this exercise is designed for self-analysis and may be done in the privacy of one's home or in private at one's desk in the class-room. However, there are other ways to use this material so that it becomes a shared rather than an individual experience. One method is to ask six people in the class to leave the room. Then flash the illustration on a screen (an opaque projector in a darkened room is suitable). Have the class discuss for two or three minutes what is happening in the scene.

Then ask one person of the six outside to come in and look at the scene. He is instructed that he will tell the next person to be called in what is happening in the picture. (The rest of the class must be very quiet during this whole process. It may be suggested that they take notes on how the story changes as it is told and re-told.)

When the first person has looked at the picture for as long as he wishes to, then it is taken off the screen. One person at a time is called into the room and is told the story by the preceding person. The last person tells it to the whole class.

Then the class discusses the changes they have detected in the telling. Often these changes reflect the feelings and beliefs of the storytellers. A group is able—without accusing an individual of distortion or attacking him for his error—to see how experiences in our kind of society affect the way we see one another. Prejudices that were originally denied become apparent, fears that have never been put into words before become apparent, and the complacency that accompanies lack of awareness is dissipated.

SEXISM IN NURSING

Though women nurses often seem to feel that there is something not quite natural about men in nursing, they deal with the men in the profession in a curiously paradoxical way. Succumbing to their own second-class status in society, the women in the profession apparently believe that men have greater natural ability for supervision and administration. (How often have we heard women say, "I *hate* working for a woman! I'd rather work for a man any day!) And so the victims of prejudice and discrimination, given the option to change the pattern, unwittingly become agents for perpetuating it!

Other groups involved in the total picture of health care demonstrate a variety of attitudes related to sex. These attitudes, taken together, seem to reinforce the pattern of prejudice and discrimination operating primarily to the disadvantage of women and sometimes to the disadvantage of men. (Nor do the two sets of disadvantages cancel each other!)

For example, patients assigned to a male nurse have been known to refuse his help, insisting that a "real nurse" be sent to them. Also, although women patients will usually accept a male physician, more of them will reject a male nurse. Male patients not infrequently view a male nurse with a lurking suspicion that his choice of profession somehow reflects adversely on his masculinity.

Women nurses very often say that they prefer men to women as patients. They maintain women are fussier, more complaining, more demanding of personal services that intrude unreasonably on the time and efforts of nurses, and less appreciative of those services than men are. The effect of this is to perpetuate the stereotype of the dependent, childish, individual, over-concerned with self. (Interestingly enough, similar behavior in men is viewed with humorous tolerance as rather appealing. "Oh, men are such babies!" women smile, in motherly superiority!) Even if it is true that women are this way (and I seriously doubt that it is), then it behooves the professional in any field to examine the causes of such behavior and to deal with it in productive ways, rather than to use it as justification for disliking and avoiding the client.

The attitude of men toward women in our society, and the corresponding attitude of men physicians toward women nurses, is also part of the picture. Despite the accomplishments of women—often in the face of systematic discrimination—the error persists that women are intellectually inferior to men. When men have doubts about their own adequacy, they cling to this picture of women that helps them feel superior by comparison. This attitude is apparent in the comments of many male physicians who suggest that women cannot measure a dose of medicine accurately, or read a chart and follow the directions without making some kind of dumb mistake. Of course, like most bigots, they insist that they are not prejudiced, because they can always point to one nurse who is a "gem," *one* capable woman who "runs the place"—whatever the place happens to be. (As I say, every bigot has his "exception.")

Physicians with such attitudes toward women nurses may be partly responsible for the practice of limiting the medical knowledge of nurses ("Why do they have to know causes of disease?") and consequently limiting their ability to make professional judgments ("They're just supposed to follow the doctor's orders."). Even many of the women in nursing have traditionally accepted this limitation of the nurse's role, so the current struggle to operate as equals on the health team is waged not only with men but also with women as antagonists.

This is not uncharacteristic of minority-group people. Reared in a dominating society that treats them as inferiors, they often grow up with some vestige of belief that they really *are* inferior. With women this belief becomes apparent in the whole pattern of relationships between men and women in our society. Women often do not prepare for jobs that are traditionally seen as men's jobs for fear of being thought unfeminine. They accommodate themselves to the common business pattern of the male executive with a constellation of capable females in his orbit. (This pattern is not seen in reverse, with a woman executive and a group of men in tow.) And they are forever fearful of being condemned as over-aggressive for demonstrating the drive and ambition for which men are rewarded.

With men physicians and women nurses self-denigration takes the form of deferring to the doctor's point of view (even if that point of view is not substantiated by greater knowledge), hesitating to object to a physician's behavior that is not in the best interest of the patient, and being reluctant to broaden the nurse's medical expertise and judgment. I have even seen a woman nurse stand up when a male physician came into the room!

In other more subtle ways, the lower status of women continues to be perpetuated. I have heard physicians maintain that nurse's aides were more effective nurses than RNs were. Their feeling was that aides offered a patient more warmth, empathy, and a human kind of reaching out than did RNs. You will notice that the approved qualities are consistent with the stereotype of a woman—there is nothing in them of professional expertise or efficiency. The ideal nurse, for them, is one who has had little or no professional training and whose capabilities are those that a woman "should" have—and that might be seen as weakness in a man. With this kind of evaluation of nursing practice, the woman is subtly assigned to her place—because she's so perfect for that place!

Try this small experiment and bring back your findings to discuss with your colleagues in class. For one whole day, no matter what activity you are engaged in, watch and listen for evidences of sexist attitudes and behaviors. Each time you hear someone say something, see someone do something, or read something that is sexist, make a quick note of it. (Don't forget the jokes and the wisecracks with women as the target! Humor is a very effective way to cloak prejudice.)

Before you meet with your class, re-copy the evidence in two columns, Column 1 for those items that you discovered outside of nursing, and Column 2 for those that deal specifically with nursing. See if you can find some connections between the items in Column 1 and those in Column 2. For example, suppose you see a newspaper that quotes a man as saying, about the Women's Liberation Movement, "All right! They want to be like men, let them! But watch a woman complain when I don't stand up and give her my seat or I don't hold a door for her!" This goes in Column 1, as an example of how prejudice obscures one's ability to perceive the goals of the movement accurately. An item in Column 2 might be the remark of a male physician who retorts when a female nurse complains about being overworked, "You want equality! Well, stop complaining!" Again an apparent distortion caused by the animosity that is usually an integral part of prejudice.

In a class of thirty people, you should amass an interesting collection of data. The purpose of this exercise is twofold: (1) The first step in dealing with any problem is becoming aware of its existence. Often, reared in a society with a pervasive social problem, we absorb that problem into our total way of life and are not even aware of its existence or the damage it causes. (2) The next step in dealing with such a problem is expressing our feelings about it. Anger, frustration, and annoyance that are suppressed or even pushed out of our consciousness are inevitably displaced to destructive uses. Unable to express our feelings about the real problem, we may vent them on innocent targets or make ourselves ill. (3) The third step entails obtaining as much data as we can about the causes of the problem and attempts that have been made to solve it in our lives and in our areas of operation.

Sharing what you have discovered and expressing your feelings about it all is better done in small groups of eight or nine people rather than in a whole class. In this way, everyone will have the opportunity to speak and, in the relative privacy of the small group, be encouraged to express feelings they might be reluctant to express in a large group. Let me say just another word here about group discussion. We have a myth in education called "class discussion." Actually, there is no such thing. What teachers do when they have a "class discussion" is engage in a conversation with five or six people in the class while the rest just look on. If discussion is indeed an integral and valuable part of the learning process, then optimum opportunity must be provided for it for every student. The small group is a way of making such provision. This does not, however, mean that students invariably know how to use this opportunity to the best advantage. Teachers may need to help them learn discussion skills. Since working in groups to solve problems is a widespread practice, it might be worthwhile to take the time to learn those skills even in a class in nurse-patient relationships.[1]

Gathering additional factual material on the causes and attempted cures of sexism may also be done on a small-group basis, with the work being divided among the various members who then come back together to share what they have learned. Material may be gathered from books and periodicals, from interviewing people who have worked in the field, from government agencies, employment agencies, and any other sources that you may discover.

The first steps in attempting to solve the problems occur in the relatively safe atmosphere of the classroom, utilizing such techniques as role-playing and systematic exploration of alternative solutions, which we shall deal with in Chapter 3.

AGE AND PREJUDICE: STEREOTYPING THE GENERATIONS

Stereotyping is such an habitual mode of thinking in our society that we find it operating wherever people come into interaction with one another. In the discussion after the game, *The Ideal Nurse and Patient,* it often becomes clear that such traits as open-mindedness and ability to accept new ideas are clearly associated with young people. The feeling seems to be that as soon as people reach a certain age—twenty? twenty-five? —they begin to build a wall around what they have already learned and become more and more insulated against new ideas and new ways of doing things.

This perception of advancing age reminds me of a belief I had as a child. Reared as I was in a city neighborhood where most of the parents were Jewish immigrants, I was aware that, although the children spoke English, the older people usually spoke Yiddish or English with an accent. At the age of five or six I thought that as a person grew into maturity, he forgot how to speak English and used only Yiddish to communicate.

[1] Again, see my book, *Affective Subjects* . . . for the "Four Stage Rocket" that teaches small-group discussion skills.

I think we must look a little more closely at the problems that are apparent between older and younger nurses and see if we cannot isolate the errors in our perception of one another. The picture of the ideal nurse as young, and the open-minded, forward-looking, *middle-aged* nurse as an exception to the general rule is neither accurate nor helpful in developing productive relationships.

When student nurses come on to the hospital floor, they often expect to see the older nurses using archaic practices, and they have a tendency to attribute most difficulties of interaction to age differences. Actually, the different expectations of nursing service personnel and nursing education personnel make up the fertile ground in which the stereotype of age flourishes. Nursing education staff is primarily responsible for seeing to it that students get the variety and depth of experience that will eventually make them effective nurses. Nursing service people are primarily concerned with seeing to it that patients get the best possible care. A student is taught certain procedures and told to use them on the floor; a working nurse or supervisor may evaluate the procedure in terms of time and staff available and number of patients to be cared for and decide that the procedure is not appropriate. Then begins the tug-of-war between nursing education and nursing service with the student's behavior as the prize—is the student to do what is "right," what is *clinically* appropriate, or what is seen as "practical?" As this scene repeats itself throughout the student's training period, it is not difficult for the young person to conclude that after you have been around for a while, after you have been a nurse for a number of years, you are set in your ways and no change is accomplished without resistance and antagonism from the older nurses.

Thus, new nurses coming into a hospital *expect* older nurses to resist change and refuse to accept the new knowledge that young people bring with them. The older nurses expect young people to reject all that the more experienced people have learned in the course of their careers. It is these *expectations* that interfere with communication and cooperation. The *facts* are that young nurses are not universally ready to use what is new, nor are older nurses always so set on holding on to what is old. Rather, both groups are more caught up in maintaining their conceptions of themselves and one another.

The pervasive attitude toward older people that characterizes our society is, of course, reflected in the nursing profession in other ways. For example, the occasional older person who decides to become a nurse encounters all kinds of difficulties. Beyond a certain age, no school will accept her. The refusal is bolstered by all kinds of high-sounding and "practical" reasons, ranging all the way from waning intellectual ability with advancing age to the inadvisability of investing the time and money in professional training when the graduate will have such a relatively short time left to practice. These reasons ignore the evidence that experience and motivation more than offset whatever disability (if, indeed there is *any*) in intellect that comes with aging. And they ignore, also, the possibility that in five years of practice a fifty-five-year-old professional may make a discovery that could revolutionize the profession!

But the sad fact is that, when an older nurse is permitted to enter a program, she is continually beset with self-doubt about her ability to keep up, a self-doubt that is rarely allayed by the faculty or her fellow students. A clue to her feelings is her constant joking: "What can you expect, at my age?" and a clue to the similar feelings of the younger students is their weak smiles everytime they hear such a joking reference to her age.

PROMOTING INTERACTION

One way of getting through the barrier of the stereotype to the real person underneath is systematically to chip away at that barrier by sustained interaction. Initially, such interaction may seem forced and artificial, but, really, that is what schools are designed for—to arrange opportunities for learning. An element of artificiality is implicit in the very idea. We rarely object to the artificiality of learning about patient care out of books in the classroom, but when anyone suggests learning about people by arranging opportunities for human interaction in the class room, the specter of artificiality rears it head!

Because establishing relationships with new people is not an easy thing to do, we have a tendency to maintain already-established relationships and move only reluctantly to speak to people we do not know. In addition, the stereotypic expectations we have of other groups are often unpleasant. Consequently, in a classroom or work situation, we are most likely to make contact with people we have known from other situations, people we can identify as most like us and people who make overtures to us or seem more approachable. The result is that small cliques develop. When problems arise, the cliques easily come into conflict, because the social distance among them has inhibited communication and understanding.

To begin to encourage a different pattern of interaction in the classroom, make a decision to culminate each activity by talking over your observations with someone in the class that you do not know. Approach someone from a different age group, a different racial group, the other sex—someone you have not had occasion to interact with before. The class, then, can become a practice ground for trying out behaviors that can be used in the hospital.

Since the direction to seek out someone you don't know is a class activity, it is somewhat safer to risk oneself than it is on the outside. If rebuffed, one can always shrug off responsibility for making the overture. However, in the process people begin to realize that it is not, after all, quite so risky a venture as they imagined. People are really not so quick to rebuff overtures. So you begin to communicate with one another across all the lines set up by our society: race, sex, age, appearance, manner. The common experience of the class activity that has preceded the communication eases the first moments of strangeness. An air of friendliness begins to develop in the class. And the strength derived from being part of a group of accepting, friendly people carries us through the difficulties of initiating communication in the work situation.

The problem census, the game, and the new-contact activity all contribute to changing materially the climate of the traditional classroom. Students begin to see that they, too, have the ability—and responsibility— to take an active part in their own professional education. They no longer feel trapped in the old spoon-feeding process of education they knew as children. Instructors begin to adjust their roles, too, to a new perception of the student as first-class citizen—involved, interested, and excited about this first step on the road to a new career.

3 DEALING WITH STEREOTYPES: SIMULATING PROBLEM SITUATIONS

DEVELOPING SELF-INSIGHT

If nurses expect themselves to behave and think in ways that are in the aggregate unrealistic, and if patients have expectations of nurses that are not only unrealistic but border on the outrageous, then the questions arise: How are we to deal with these unrealistic expectations? What can we do, not only to explode the myths, but also to prevent them from interfering with our professional—and human—effectiveness? This is the thrust of most of the responses nurses make to problem census questions: Other people do this or that: What can I do to make the situation better? What should I say to the patient? How can I deal with sexism? Should a nurse make excuses? And so on, and on.

There are very few pat answers to these questions. There is no rule book that one can pull out in the face of prejudice or discrimination and find in it standard procedures for reducing prejudice or eliminating discrimination. Even if someone else told you exactly what he did, you might discover when you took his advice that you simply could not replicate the behavior. Have we not all imagined ourselves responding heroically, or firmly, or differently than we did when faced with the real thing?

However, there are ways of becoming more aware of how your feelings and behaviors might be affected by different situations, so that you are not caught completely off guard when you actually find yourself interacting with people and faced with the necessity for responding to prejudice, discrimination, conflict, hostility, fear, and confusion. By participating in the following activities, you are engaging, in a relatively safe atmosphere, in the experiences that will prepare you for actual reality testing. Here you look closely at yourself with the help of your colleagues. Then you try out your reactions in some simulated situations, examining each reaction in the light of its consequences and your own objectives. Later (Chapter 8), you can begin to replicate those reactions in real-life situations, where errors cannot so easily be erased. But by then you will be making far fewer errors because you are so much more skillful in interaction!

Groups of eight to ten students discuss the question: What are the results, in your own behavior and feelings, when people expect that you are something you are not? Very often, it is the Black students in the group who know immediately how to respond to this question. They know when people are waiting for them to be lazy, waiting to pounce on a real or imagined oversight in the performance of some task. The young Black woman who never forgot the white teacher who expressed speechless amazement at her academic ability still feels surrounded by the expectation that she is "naturally" inferior intellectually.

Then the others begin to speak, telling of their experiences with people who saw them, not as individuals, but as cardboard figures stamped out of a pattern. The long-haired man whose application for admission to a nursing program is rejected on the grounds that he does not fit the picture of a "professional"; the young woman with a twisted spine who is told that she could never "keep up" in nursing—although she has been "keeping up" at scrubbing floors and caring for three brothers and sisters for ten of her nineteen years; the gray-haired woman whom everyone expects to take the conventional, traditional side of each discussion; the pretty blonde who, it is assumed, doesn't have a serious thought in her head. All of these people begin to share, not only their experiences, but their feelings. They begin to talk about how they have had to respond to such expectations.

In one class of student nurses, the groups compiled lists of the various ways in which people said they responded in the face of stereotypic expectations. One person said that he tried to be everything people expected him to be—good or bad. Another person confessed to feeling somewhat confused, feeling that she must be doing something wrong although she started out thinking she was doing a good job. She lost her self-confidence, she said, when she realized people were seeing her as "one of those people who got their job just because of her race." One person became defensive and was forever being accused of having a chip on his shoulder. Another admitted to profound depression when he encountered this kind of prejudice, and spent a good part of his energy sedulously avoiding similar situations. And through all his avoidance strategies he

was obsessed with the conviction that there must be something wrong
with him.

Some people said that negative expectations interfered with their
efficiency generally; others were reluctant to make decisions, even when
they were objectively competent to make them. They were more worried
about the image they were trying to project in order to destroy the stereotype
than they were about the welfare of the patient. Some people got very
angry; some felt helpless and frustrated; some were only nervous and
miserable. The feeling of alienation from others was strong in some people
—especially alienation from members of other groups. Many just felt
an overwhelming sadness.

And then there were the hostile ones, who hit back at the world
that refused to see them as real people, individuals in their own right.
Many pretended, played a role that got them what they wanted while they
sneered inwardly at the bigots. Others vowed to get everything they could
from a world that gave them nothing without a fight.

One said, "I'm just myself. They can take me or leave me, but
that's what I am." Another said, "I try hard to be as professional and
carefully objective as possible when I know that a patient expects me to be
deficient in some way. I try even harder to please such a patient—partly
to prove he's wrong, but partly because I'm scared he'll prove out right."
One pretends a self-confidence she doesn't feel; another feels that all she
has to do is prove herself and the negative expectations will fade away.
The Black woman is moved to excel at everything academic and suffers
tortures that she can never achieve perfection. The long-haired man views
the "establishment" as the enemy and looks to resist it even when he sees
it doing something of which he approves. The overworked young woman
becomes bitter and miserable; the older woman defensive and resentful.
And the pretty blonde shrugs her shoulders and makes her own way. All of
them begin to see that their experiences have really not been so very
different, that they have much in common. Although they have begun by
seeing themselves as separated by wide gulfs, they now begin to understand
one another and feel for one another. They are not so far apart as they
thought they were!

The next step is to consider what assumptions *they* make about
the people with whom they interact, what beliefs and feelings *they* have
about whole groups of people that they identify and catalogue in groups on
the basis of a single trait.

How does one become aware that, despite his protestations that he
treats every person as an individual, he is in reality reacting to people in
terms of group stereotypes? Do you remember the nursing student who
thought nurses were disembodied virtues? Do you remember the patient

who thought all nurses were white? These individuals also believed that they approached each person as an individual, expecting only the usual human traits and making no judgment until that individual revealed *his* traits. However, our society holds so strongly to the stereotypic pictures of certain groups that we often accept them without question as true. Should someone point out that these pictures are false, based on misconceptions of whole groups of people, we may scramble to find reasons to prove the pictures accurate. (After all, would *we* believe something that is not true?)

Let us look for a moment at the stereotypes our society holds of various groups. For example, let us look at two groups that have engaged in endless strife, with one group relegated to second-class citizenship and the other struggling with self-doubt and anxiety to maintain an unrealistic ideal: women and men.

Let the instructor (or a member of your group) put up on the chalkboard this chart:

Men	Women

As people in the class call out the traits that our society thinks men have—the "manly" traits—the teacher writes them in the appropriate column. The same is done with the traits our society says are characteristically women's. When you have finished this activity, you will have an idea of the stereotypes of men and women.

Just what is the stereotype that men hold of women in our society? They are emotional, mechanically inept, have no head for figures or science, want to be protected, are weak, talkative, illogical, bad drivers, catty, and they don't like men but do want to be mothers.

And what is the stereotype of men? They are logical, natural mechanics, good at math and science, masterful and protective, strong, silent, logical, good drivers, fair and open in their dealings with one another, big babies when they are not feeling well, and sexually stimulated by almost every woman who floats into their field of vision.

You may protest that everybody does not believe the stereotypes, and of course you are right. However, enough people hold them so that businesses and institutions often operate as if they were true. Women have difficulty being accepted in professions like law and engineering. Advertisements encourage men to "promise her anything" with the implication that promises to "her" are not to be taken seriously. Tax laws do not recognize child care as a legitimate deductible expense for working mothers.

The interesting thing about stereotypes is that the group that is victimized by a society often begins to believe the stereotype too. If, all around us, people, the media, and institutions seem to operate on the premise that the traits of the stereotype are accurate, then the victim begins to think that there *must* be some truth in the picure. Even though she is certain that the picture in that right-hand column is not of *her,* she believes that it must accurately describe all those other members of her group; and she *may actually reject* that part of her that must inevitably be identified with her fellow group members. The individual who does this may actually dislike himself—a condition that is anxiety-producing and destructive.

Similarly, we might look at the stereotypes of two other groups, also embattled, with one group virtually destroyed by the consequences of prejudice and discrimination.

What Whites Think Blacks Are Like	What Blacks Think Whites Are Like
dirty	rich
lazy	they have it made—all opportunities
smell bad	are available to them
violent	can't dance
happy-go-lucky	sexually deficient
all alike	the men want Black women
have rhythm	are physical cowards
good dancers	are hypocrites, especially in relation
drunks	to the rights of Black people
the men want white women	all alike
criminals	feel superior
more powerful sexually	
make rotten soldiers	
intellectually inferior	

Given this picture that men have of women and women of men, and that Blacks and whites have of each other, what would one think they *feel* about one another? Write the feelings in the narrow column between the stereotypes. How *do* you feel about someone you believe is over-emotional, illogical, and inept in a number of significant ways? How do you feel about someone you believe is everything that you are not or never can be? How do you feel about someone you believe is dirty, lazy and violent—or hypocritical and supercilious? The chances are that your feelings toward one another will reflect your beliefs: You will dislike, distrust, and resent one another. At the very least, you will avoid equal contact; at the other extreme, you may kill one another. If there were no benefit in exploitation (in the one case, sex is often used in an exploitative way; in the other, exploitation is more often economic), the groups would probably avoid one another completely.

The barrier of feelings among the groups actually prevents equal-status communication. We see one another through a haze of negative emotions, and the result is that the distortions are increased and reinforced. Finally, we do not know how to get through this barrier in order to see one another as whole human beings very much like ourselves.

Do doctors and nurses hold stereotypes of each other that impede effective communication between them? No? What about male doctors and female nurses? And male nurses and female doctors? Given the male/female stereotypes in our society, it is likely that they become apparent in doctor-nurse interaction too! But aside from that problem, do doctors and nurses have one-dimensional distorted pictures of each other that are directly related to their professional functions? I have seen evidence that they do.

There is the story of the physician who was called in by the director of a nursing program to lecture to a group of students on the topic of allergies. The doctor spoke for about an hour and then turned to leave. The director walked after him to thank him again for coming. "Incidentally, doctor," she observed, "I noticed that while you recounted in great detail the symptoms and care of allergic reactions, you never went into the causes of allergy."

The doctor turned on her with some annoyance, "What the hell are you trying to do," he said, "make doctors of these nurses?"

The implication was clear: Nurses don't need reasons for what they do. Theirs is only to take doctor's orders!

There are physicians who look with some skepticism on the long periods of professional education designed for nurses. They feel that nurses do not need to know much, and that they can tell a nurse all she needs to do her job in a few days of on-the-job training. Some even go on to say that they prefer LPNs and aides to RNs, because the LPNs and aides really know how to do the necessary nursing job, with little technical knowledge but much warmth and unquestioning obedience to the doctor's wishes.

And then there is the nurse who is afraid to call a doctor's attention to an error. What is the cause of the fear? It may be a fear of reprisal, because the doctor is powerful enough to remove anyone who dares to question the correctness of his behavior. Is there a stereotype involved here? Are all doctors really so touchy about their errors, or is this just a part of the picture nurses have of them? Do nurses believe that doctors are inevitably more right than nurses are, just because they are doctors? But what about the nurse's professional province? Aren't there some things she knows more about than doctors do? Perhaps the fear is partly a function of the separation between doctors and nurses, the psychological distance, the lack of equal-status communication. Through the barriers of misunderstanding and resentment that separate them, the stereotype looms as menacing. Are doctors also afraid of nurses?

EXPLORING ALTERNATIVE SOLUTIONS

Given our errors in the way we perceive one another, the chances are that we are sometimes less than effective when we find ourselves in problem situations with one another. Unfortunately—or perhaps fortunately for our continuing humanity—no one can give us a collection of problems involving human interaction and step-by-step instructions on how to solve them. Nor can we afford to wait until we encounter a problem to try out a variety of solutions until we happen on the right one: the insensitive words, the impulsive behavior may destroy all possibility for communication forever, and eliminate all chances for trying out other words or other behaviors.

What we can do is simulate situations and, in the relative safety of simulation, test out alternative ways of dealing with them. Here, if we say something that causes anger or do something that makes a person avoid us, we can always backtrack and try again, this time with different results. When the time comes that we are involved in a similar situation in real life, we are ready with a number of possible ways of behaving and some idea of how each way affects others. Still, there are no absolute assurances of success, for no two situations are exactly alike. However, the possibility of gross error is substantially reduced.

There are a number of ways of using simulation to test out solutions. The one I have found most helpful is role-playing. In this technique we take a familiar situation that presents a problem or conflict of some kind, right up to but not including the first step in dealing with the conflict. Then we ask, what happens now? Instead of then *discussing* the various possibilities, people in the class assume the roles of the different characters in the situation and continue the story by actually acting it out. When the role players have taken the solution as far as they can (they should not spend more than about ten minutes at this), everyone discusses what happened: how people felt in the situation and what behaviors elicited what responses.

Then the questions are raised: Are there other ways of dealing with this situation? Are there other responses we might want to elicit from the people involved? The situation is then re-played with role players who want to try alternative behaviors. After the role-playing, the class again discusses what happened and the consequences of the actions taken. The situation may be re-played as often as the class wishes, so that every possible action may be examined in the light of the consequences. Just which mode of action an individual selects when faced with the real-life situation is, of course, his own concern. However, he is now equipped to make a choice on the basis of what he has learned about the consequences of that choice. His action need not be impulsive or blind.

In the next section, a number of situations are presented that are useful for role-playing. Students should take on the roles at the point at which I ask: What happens now? Do not read the discussion that follows this question until you have had an opportunity to explore some of your own solutions.

TEN SITUATIONS FROM LIFE AND SOME TENTATIVE SOLUTIONS

1. *"You're an exception."* Cindy Brown is planning to enter the professional nursing program at the University in September. Now, in June, she has a job in a small hospital as a nurse's aide. At dinner one evening she is sitting in the hospital cafeteria with several other hospital employees. As usual, the topic of discussion is the patients they are all caring for.

One aide sitting next to Cindy starts to talk about an old Jewish woman she has as a patient, and how she expects all her demands to be met without question. "She thinks you ought to stay with her for all eight hours of the shift!" the aide says. "She wants to have a private duty nurse when she goes home in a couple of days. Cheap Jew, she'll probably give you a dollar an hour and have you work your rear off. And I know she has money!" Suddenly, something occurs to the aide and she turns to Cindy. "You're not Jewish, are you?" "Yes, I am," says Cindy. "Oh, you don't look like one. Anyway, you're different from the others."

What happens now?

Feelings   First, let us conjecture about the feelings of the people in this situation. Cindy Brown may feel very angry at this evidence that Jewish people are held in contempt by her co-worker, for the contempt does include her too, despite the denial that she is "different." Inasmuch as she is Jewish, the condemnation of Jews inevitably touches her.

Does the denial make her feel more or less angry? Curiously, she feels ambivalent about it. In a society that expresses and acts out anti-Semitic attitudes, it may be somewhat comforting to be told that the attitudes are not directed against you personally. Too, the self-doubt often generated by prejudice may move one to find comfort even in this left-handed kind of compliment. (The self-doubt arises when minority-group children grow up in a world that takes pains to make it clear that the child's group is undesirable in a number of very specific ways. Although each member of the group may, on one level, be sure that the prejudice is based on misconceptions about his group, it is sometimes difficult to escape some flicker of doubt and fear that the stereotype contains an element of truth. We even have proverbs to lend credence to these feelings: "Fifty-million Frenchmen can't be wrong," and "Where there's smoke there's fire." We are taught quite effectively that these proverbs are true, but how many teachers ever take the time to teach that a stereotype is a lie? This is a "proverb" with much more validity than most of the others we learn!)

Does Cindy feel hurt when she hears the anti-Semitic sentiment expressed? Does she feel like crying at this evidence of wholesale rejection of her group?

And what of the other aide? Is she embarrassed that her attitude was expressed in the company of a Jew? Does she habitually reserve her expressions of prejudice for those times when she is only with her own group? Or is she quite comfortable in her conviction that she is right, especially since everyone else at the table seems to have accepted what she said.

The other people at the table? They are embarrassed, so they just change the subject. Or they dislike the aide for being an anti-Semite. Or they agree with her and are pleased that someone had the guts to say what should have been said.

Alternative behaviors   What would happen if Cindy said to the aide, "I'm really not different. Can't you see that I have horns growing out of my head?" What would this expression of anger accomplish? It might make Cindy feel good that she was able to express her anger so freely. It might make the aide aware of the effect of her anti-Semitism. Or it might only make the aide angry and reinforce her hostile feelings toward Jews.

How about the other people at the table? How would it affect them? Would they think twice about expressing prejudice in public? Would they dislike Cindy for being so "touchy?" Would they admire her for standing up for herself so bravely? Would they voice their approval for putting a bigot in her place?

Any of these are possibilities, and, of course, we never know when we choose a course of action just exactly what the results will be. However, the individual who has tried out a number of different behaviors feels more confident that, when he does make a choice, the effect does not hit him with completely unexpected force.

2. *"I hate all of them."* Annette Berger is an RN on the medical-surgical floor of Blank Hospital. One day, her aunt is brought in for minor surgery, and Annette sits for a few minutes talking to her. Then, hoping to help establish a friendly atmosphere in the two-bed room, she draws the other patient into the conversation. "Mrs. Jaret," she says, "Why don't you sit up a little more, so you can be more comfortable?"

Before Annette knows what's happening, Mrs. Jaret is yelling at her. "I'm not taking any orders from you! All you Germans think the whole world has to do what you tell it to! Well, this is America, and you Germans aren't the master race!"

Now what happens?

Feelings   What is Mrs. Jaret feeling? Has she suffered personally at the hands of the Nazis? Perhaps the fear of her illness is coming out as anger, and whatever feeling she may have had about Germans is used as a vehicle to focus that anger. Perhaps her outburst surprised even herself, because she has never before lashed out at strangers this way. Perhaps she has even prided herself on being free from the usual prejudices. Or perhaps she really is extremely prejudiced and hates all Germans— and anyone else who is different from herself.

And Annette? Has she experienced similar attacks from others, or is this a new experience for her? How does *she* feel about being German? Has she thought much about what the Nazis did and has she felt some guilt herself? Or does she feel that, since she was not living during the Hitler era, she has no responsibility for what happened then?

Is she angry that someone accuses her of something she had nothing to do with? Is she worried at the effect of all this on her sick aunt?

Perhaps this is an old story to Annette's aunt. She came to the United States after the Second World War and people did confront her with hostility and rejection. How had she dealt with this in the past? Was she angry that people blamed her for what the German government did? Did she feel guilty that, as a German citizen, she did nothing to protest the persecution and killings? Does she insist to this day that she knew nothing of what was going on? Or does she maintain that the past should be forgotten and that people should just get on with the business of living?

Alternative behaviors   Does Annette just keep silent with surprise and shock? Does she say to herself, "This woman is sick; I mustn't agitate her any more by reacting with anger?" Does Annette's aunt feel moved to come to her niece's defense—and to her own because she is

German too? Is there, perhaps, something to be gained by taking Mrs. Jaret's hand and assuring her that no one was giving her orders (and then, perhaps in a quieter moment, exploring with her the belief that not all people of German background are Nazis)? How would Mrs. Jaret respond if Annette just pulled the curtain between the beds and isolated her—and her aunt too, in the bargain? What are all the possible consequences of all the possible behaviors?

3. *"Everybody knows what they're like."* Jim Lawrence and John Demron were hitching a ride home from the University. A station wagon stopped, and the driver, a white, middle-aged man, told them to get in. Jim sat in the back, John beside the driver, and a conversation started. The driver asked them what they did, and they told him that they were freshman nursing students at Blank Hospital. His response was, "You must see a lot of gunshot wounds and stabbing cases working in *that* neighborhood." (The hospital is located in the middle of a poor black neighborhood in the heart of the city.)

Jim and John told him that, contrary to his opinion, most of the patients admitted were not suffering from gunshot and stabbing wounds. He flushed—in embarrassment or anger—and became insistent: "I'm sure Friday and Saturday nights are the busiest in the emergency wards. All the drunkards and niggers walking around."

John turned and looked out the window. Jim shrank into the back seat with a look of disgust on his face. Now what happens?

Feelings   The real Jim to whom it happened felt greatly depressed at the driver's attitude. He felt that it was useless to contradict him, because he seemed so set in his way of thinking. (The word Jim actually used was "worthless". It was worthless to contradict him, he said.) Did he really feel that the man himself was worthless? Is that why he did not bother to make the effort to help him change? The real John confessed that he hadn't liked the man the minute he'd got into the car, and this attitude only reinforced his dislike. However, he felt that, since he was a passenger in the man's car, he was not able to express his own opinion freely. Out of gratitude for the lift? (Is honesty really so completely dependent on appreciation for a small favor?) Out of fear that he would be put out of the car? Out of fear that the driver would become so disturbed in the face of a contradiction that his driving would endanger them all?

Alternative behaviors   What would you do in this situation? How far would you risk yourself psychologically by exposing yourself to anger and hostility or physically by exposing yourself to a crazy driver?

And once you took the risk, is it possible that you would encounter no danger at all? Is it possible that the driver would shut up, chagrined at finding that everyone does not share his sentiments? (What a salutary thing to learn—that the whole world doesn't agree with you! If you can really teach someone this, you are not doing them a disservice. On the contrary, it is a favor that brings them a step closer to mental health.)

You might give him additional information about the patients in the hospital and so provide raw material for reconsideration of his point of view. You might offer him a tour of the hospital, so that he can check out the information for himself. (Incidentally, he might meet some patients and begin to see them as real people, suffering from the same ills as everyone else.) Of course, you might tell him he's an ignorant old fool, and that he doesn't know what he's talking about. What do you think his response to *that* would be?!

Is it possible that the silence of Jim and John misled him into believing that they were agreeing with him? Silence often is interpreted in this way. People think that those who are silent have no countering arguments, do not really believe the person is wrong, or at least do not believe it strongly enough to say something. Do you think Jim and John really wanted the driver to leave, believing something like this about them?

4. *"I've got to do it all myself."* Miss Smith, the charge nurse, walks about with a perpetual air of being put upon. She's a hard and skillful worker and does not hesitate to make a bed or answer a bell if the LPNs are busy. But she has said a number of times that nursing care has deteriorated since LPNs and aides have replaced the scarce RNs at bedside care and that the only way she can be sure patients get what they need is for her to take over some of the duties herself. She is sure no LPN has enough professional commitment to be concerned about whether or not the patient is getting adequate care. As a matter of fact, she is sure that, even when they are *told* what to do, they follow the orders only minimally and get away with as much as they can.

One day, an LPN hears Miss Smith say—in her usual martyred way—"Those people! They just can't be depended on to do what has to be done. I supposed I'd better get in there and see to it, or it will never get done."

Miss Camacho, the LPN, turns to Miss Smith angrily.
What does she say?

Feelings   Miss Camacho was obviously very angry. She probably perceived the phrase "those people" as the kind of denigrating epithet so often used about minority-group people. (She was of Mexican background and no stranger to victimization of this kind.) Miss Smith is startled and dismayed at Miss Camacho's anger. She probably has grown so accustomed to her own attitudes and her expression of them that she is almost unaware of the real effect they may have on the people around her. As a matter of fact, most of her co-workers do not even seem to hear her any more; they simply shrug their shoulders and go their own way. But Miss Smith does not know what they are thinking.

What might their thoughts be—the Black and Puerto Rican and Mexican LPNs and aides? Perhaps they think, "If she's so sure she's the only one who does the job, then let her do it." And they do as little as possible (and Miss Smith becomes the one who *causes* what she's always complaining about).

Some people might think: "These Anglos, these whites! *They're* all alike. They'll fault you no matter how hard you work, so why should we break our necks?" One person does just about "break her neck" and never gets a word of recognition or encouragement from Miss Smith.

And what of Miss Smith? Does she really believe what she is saying? If she were pinned down and asked: "Do you actually believe that all aides are lazy and stupid?" What would her answer be? I think she would deny believing this. Perhaps she would only go so far as to say that *most* were this way. Perhaps she might get a flash of self-insight and recognize what was really motivating her attitude. Perhaps she would have to admit—if only to herself—that she had so great a need to prove to the world that she was doing a magnificent job and that her need was so mixed up with her feelings of self-doubt that she could feel successful only by seeing everyone else as a failure. Is this kind of self-insight too much to expect of anyone? Well, maybe a colleague could help Miss Smith see it.

Alternative behaviors   Suppose that Miss Camacho shouted at Miss Smith, "Who do you think you are? What gives you the right to talk that way about us? You think you're so perfect, so wonderful? You have no right to insult people!"

How would Miss Smith react? Would she deny that she was insulting anyone? Would she retreat in fear and later emerge expressing anger and indignation at how *those people* talked to her? Would her attitude simply be reinforced, or would she begin to realize the debilitating effect it had on people and how she was destroying morale?

Suppose that another RN, Miss Johns, had overheard the exchange between Miss Smith and Miss Camacho and decided to say something. Suppose that she waited until Miss Camacho had "blown her top" and stalked off before she said to Miss Smith, "You look so surprised—almost as if you surely didn't ever mean to be hurting people's feelings." How might Miss Smith answer? Maybe she would just burst into tears before she could say anything. And when the storm was over, Miss Johns could make time to sit down with Miss Smith and perhaps help her understand what

had just happened. This approach might have made an unpleasant alter-
cation a very worthwhile thing.

5. *"Let 'em learn to be Americans."* Miss Watson was a nurse
who expended great effort to establish optimal communication between
herself and her patients. After eight years of experience in a large metropolitan hospital, she had actually accumulated a small library of foreign-
language dictionaries so that she could pick up a few words in almost
any language. This helped enormously when a patient who spoke little
or no English was brought on to the floor; so much of the patient's anxiety
was alleviated when he heard a few words of reassurance in his own
language.

One day, as Miss Watson is smilingly struggling with her few words
of Spanish at the bedside of a middle-aged Puerto Rican woman who has
just been brought in, Miss Jones comes into the room. Miss Jones is a
nurse who devotes herself completely to her job. She is businesslike and
efficient and wastes no time as she goes about her duties. She does not smile
very much or make small talk and has, on at least one occasion, been
heard to say that the job of the nurse is to attend to the patient's physical
needs and nothing more.

Miss Jones stands and watches Miss Watson for a moment. She
fidgets impatiently and frowns with displeasure. Finally she bursts out,
"Why don't you stop that nonsense! Our time is too valuable to waste it on
people like this. She wants to live in the United States—let her learn
English! Why should we have to learn Spanish? English is the language of
this country!"

What happens now?

Feelings   Do you think that what Miss Jones said made Miss
Watson feel guilty? Do you think that perhaps she began to doubt the
purity of her own motives when her colleagues seemed to think she was just
wasting valuable time? Or was she so confident of the professional validity
of her objective that she was able to see Miss Jones's point of view as a
narrow and unprofessional one?

What does *really* bother Miss Jones? Is she so overworked that she
feels she must cut out everything except for bare essentials? Or does she
really believe that the patients' mental state is not the nurse's concern? Or
does she simply dislike people who are different from herself, speak
different languages, have different customs? Does she believe that people
from other countries are too lazy to learn English? Or does she think they
are so arrogant that they expect Americans to learn *their* language?

What about the patient? Is it possible that she understands enough
English to know what Miss Jones has said? Does this make her feel angry?

Hurt? Frightened at what might happen to her at the hands of unsympathetic people? Was she affected at all by Miss Watson's attempts to speak Spanish? Does she see it as an insulting assumption that she cannot understand English, or a friendly attempt to establish communication?

Alternative behaviors   Suppose that Miss Watson says to her colleague, "Will you excuse me for a few minutes, Miss Jones? I'll be finished settling Mrs. Ramirez in and then we can talk."

How do you think Miss Jones would respond to such a noncommittal, polite, but firm request? She might simply turn and walk out. She might continue her verbal attack on Miss Watson, only this time it would be directed more personally against her—a sort of "Who do you think you are to talk to me that way?" barrage.

What if Miss Watson turns to Miss Jones and says icily, "This does not concern you. I will thank you to mind your own business." Miss Jones might respond to this with, "It *is* my business if I have to do your work while you play social worker!" Or she might turn on her heel and walk out angrily and never talk to Miss Watson again. Do you think, knowing Miss Jones's commitment to encouraging communication, that she would say something that would be likely to cut off all communication?

And what might Mrs. Ramirez say? Might she say indignantly, "I am an American citizen—as good as you!" (Puerto Ricans *are* American citizens, you know. And so Spanish is the official language of a part of the United States!) Might she begin to cry and adversely affect her physical condition? Might she become agitated and try to get out of bed, saying that she wants to leave this place? What about the other patients on the floor? How will some of them react to all of this?

6. *"These poor children are not loved."* Miss Kingston is a pediatric nurse in a community health center. She really loves children and feels a great responsibility to alleviate the pain and unhappiness of every child who comes to her attention.

This day a very sick three-year-old is brought into the center by her mother. The mother looks scarcely old enough to be out of elementary school. In response to a series of rapid-fire questions from Miss Kingston, about the onset and duration of the illness, the young mother's voice gets lower and lower and finally fades away in an "I don't know" and "I don't remember." The weary shrug of her shoulders apparently angers Miss Kingston, because her voice gets louder and she is almost shouting as she says, "You were quick enough to have a baby, but now you don't care what happens to it! Don't you see she's very sick? Show some feeling for your own child!"

What happens now?

Feelings   Miss Kingston is so kind and soft-spoken with her child patients, why this hostile outpouring on the child-mother? Why does she seem to think that the mother does not care what happens to her baby? Is it possible that Miss Kingston believes—as so many do—that poverty-stricken parents have no love for their children? Does she, like many white people, think that poor Black children need—above all else—*love?* Does she have a feeling that, whereas white babies are conceived in love and generally cherished, Black babies are the result of promiscuity and are rejected as unwanted encumbrances?

Or is it that Miss Kingston resents young mothers, generally, as being irresponsible and uncaring? Does she believe that very young girls have babies they neither want nor care about and that they need constant reminders of their responsibility for the new life they've brought into the world? Does Miss Kingston sometimes feel despair that—with all the love *she* has to give—she has never had a child of her own, and now she probably never will?

Although the young mother seems apathetic, she undoubtedly has some feelings too in this situation. Is the apparent apathy really lack of interest in her child, or is she so confused and frightened by the child's illness that she is unable to respond in any other way? Has she been worried for some time about the baby's symptoms, yet only recently heard about the free care available at the health center? Is she just worn down with the responsibility for the baby, the worry about inadequate income, and the persistent feeling that she needs to make more of her life than this? (She had been told by her teachers that she was bright; she showed academic ability. She had wanted to be a teacher, once.)

Perhaps she is just shocked and surprised at the nurse's outburst. She had come here in desperation, looking for understanding and help, and she had been attacked. Perhaps this was the last straw to her burdens and she can feel a responsive anger slowly building inside her. Maybe she thinks, "This is all I could expect—another example of white prejudice."

Alternative behaviors   What if the mother suddenly bursts into tears as her fear and anger overwhelm her? Will Miss Kingston's natural feeling for others take over and will she try to comfort her? Will she feel some satisfaction at the thought that she has made the mother realize her own failings?

Perhaps the nurse will merely proceed to care for the baby and absolve herself of all responsibility for a mother who "brought this on herself."

What if the mother's anger takes over, and she berates the nurse in no uncertain terms: "Who do you think you are, talking to me that way?

Your job is to care for the sick people who come here, not to get nasty with anyone! You're all alike—you just want a chance to make people feel like dirt!" What if she clutches her child to her and runs from the center in blind anger? What does the nurse do then?

7. *"You've had your day; now relax and take it easy."* The young doctor was just finishing replacing the dressing on the old man's leg. "All right, Pop," said the doctor. "This should do it. You'll be out of here in a day or two."

The nurse saw a frown crease the patient's forehead; the doctor had already turned away, and was leaving. "Oh, doctor," the patient called, tentatively. "I'd . . . uh . . . I'd like to ask . . . will I be able to go back to work soon?"

The doctor turned back, startled. "Work?" he asked. "You still work? It's time you retired—a man your age." Then, as the patient started to answer, "I'll see you tomorrow. Take it easy, now." And he turned to leave again.

What happens now?

Feelings   What did the patient's frown mean? Did he dislike being addressed as "Pop"? Did he, perhaps, see himself as a man still able to function adequately in life, and did this form of address imply that he was relegated to a corner for the very aged? Was he being stereotyped as someone to be patronized and humored rather than seen as a sensitive, aware human being? How did he, then, feel about the doctor's assumption that he was no longer expected to work? Did he, perhaps, pride himself on his continuing ability to support himself and make a useful contribution to the world? What did the young man's assumption do for his sense of self, optimism, and his enthusiasm for life?

Did the nurse understand the patient's feelings? Had she, perhaps, had the opportunity to talk to him and so learn something about his self-concept and his life? Was she annoyed with the doctor for his lack of sensitivity? Perhaps, on the contrary, she felt exactly the same way— that people should stop working at some predetermined age. Perhaps her own career plans were being thwarted because older administrators refused to retire and give younger people a chance for advancement.

And what of the doctor's feelings? Was he really so completely unaware of the errors he was making in his perception of the patient? Can an educated man, professionally successful, still stereotype whole groups of people without a glimmer of awareness of what he is doing?

Is it possible that he feels so uncomfortable in the presence of old age that he cannot relax enough to let his sight clear?

Alternative behaviors   The patient, consistent with his apparent independence and self-confidence, may firmly stop the doctor's departure and insist that he be given a serious prognosis, rather than be put off almost playfully as if he were senile. Or, he may feel so discouraged by the doctor's attitude that he falls silent, and even seems to lose interest altogther in leaving the hospital.

The nurse may say nothing at all, absorbed in her own concerns with aging people. Or, she may intercede by telling the doctor that this patient holds down a regular nine-to-five job, and his employer would not dream of letting him retire. She may even emphasize—not very subtly—that *Mr. Brown* is ready to get back to work as soon as his leg is healed. (Not *Pop,* doctor; *Mr. Brown.*)

Will the doctor respond angrily if his stereotypes are challenged? Or will he admit that he was in error, at least in this one instance?

8. *"I'm just sick, not retarded!"* Mrs. Smith, the attractive middle-aged woman who had been admitted for extensive tests and, perhaps, exploratory surgery, was experiencing a short period of relative comfort. Jennie Marden, the RN on the floor, was helping her comb her hair and apply make-up preparatory to her husband's evening visit, and the two women were chatting amiably about their children and their homes.

Jennie handed her patient a mirror. "How's that?" she asked.

"Oh, that's fine. Thanks so much. I feel like a new person."

"It was a pleasure. This is more like a social visit than work. I really enjoy a small break like this."

"It *was* nice," Mrs. Smith mused. "You're so different from some other nurses. I sometimes get the feeling here that they think I'm not in full command of my faculties. Some of the people here treat me as if I'd left all my good sense at home. It really depresses me."

Just then, Mrs. Anders, another RN, comes into the room. She has apparently heard the last few sentences. Both Jennie Marden and Mrs. Smith know that Mrs. Anders has a tendency to treat her patients as if they were small children.

Now what happens?

Feelings   Mrs. Smith may have ambivalent feelings about being overheard. On the one hand, she is glad that Mrs. Anders finally knows how she feels. On the other hand, she is a little worried about how this will affect the quality of nursing care she will get from now on. Also, although it's a relief to express one's real feelings at last, it really is not very "nice" to hurt somebody else in the process.

Perhaps Mrs. Smith is not ambivalent at all. She may be very sorry she was overheard, and she may wish she had never said it at all.

Mrs. Marden may feel embarrassed for her colleague, or she may feel it was about time that somebody told Mrs. Anders that she was a nurse and not a den mother. Perhaps she has wondered for some time how to use the knowledge she has about the need of some nurses to keep their patients dependent.

Or Mrs. Marden may think, "Isn't that just like these patients. You knock yourself out to do everything for them and they never appreciate you!"

Mrs. Anders may consider Mrs. Smith's observation quite consistent with what she thinks about patients—They really don't know what's good for them. Or she may suddenly get an inkling of what she has been doing and feel some anxiety about it.

Alternative behaviors   Does everyone pretend that nothing was said and nothing was overheard? Does Mrs. Smith apologize to Mrs. Anders and explain that she didn't really mean what she said; or does she apologize for saying it behind her back and then proceed to explain in detail what has been bothering her?

Does Mrs. Anders leave in anger? Does she say something like, "Now, now. Let's not get upset about what isn't important, and just concentrate on getting well." Does she confess that she didn't mean to make people feel inferior—that she had a tendency to treat people she cared about as if they were her own relatives; and she cared about her patients.

Miss Marden says nothing (perhaps making a mental note that she will discuss this later with Mrs. Anders). Or Miss Marden says, "Let's not talk about it now; it's almost visiting time." Or Miss Marden observes, "This is an occupational hazard of nurses. We must forever be on guard against babying patients, especially those who neither need nor want babying."

9. *"You can tell by looking at them."* A young man of about eighteen has just been brought into the emergency room apparently suffering from acute appendicitis. He has long hair and a scraggly beard, and his clothes, although clean, are patched—albeit artfully. Dr. Jonsen, the resident, has just called Nurse Alys to help him with his examination. She leaves another patient in the room and approaches with evident distaste on her face.

"Hmph," she sniffs, making no effort to lower her voice, "another one of those hippies! They won't do a useful day's work, but they run right to the establishment for help when they need it! We ought to let them take care of themselves, if they think it's not important to work. How do they think we became doctors and nurses—by sitting around smoking pot, and worse? Worthless!"

Miss Ingram, the other nurse in the room, looks up from her work. The resident keeps on with what he's doing.

What happens now?

Feelings   Is Miss Alys merely giving voice to a generalized stereotype of bearded young men, or is she responding to a personal experience with one young man? Though she has never mentioned it, she may have a younger brother or son who has left home to live a style of life she characterizes as "hippie." Perhaps she wanted him to finish college, become a doctor or an architect, and his refusal to do so has been a profound disappointment to her.

Perhaps this is not the case at all. Perhaps she merely shares the view of young people that older people generally seem to have. From the time of Socrates, the generation in power has seen the upcoming generation as inferior to what *they* were at that age. Does Miss Alys think that all young men with beards and patched jeans are ne'er-do-wells, revolutionaries, and drug addicts? (Many adults seem to believe this.)

What about Miss Ingram? Does she share Miss Alys's beliefs? Does she have a good friend who looks very much like this young man? Or does she feel that open expression of such views has no place if patients can hear them?

How *does* the patient feel about the nurse's comments? Do they make him fearful that he may not get the help he needs, because the person in the helping role is hostile? Perhaps he has heard this sort of thing so often that he feels only mildly amused. Or maybe he's bitter, because this is the same kind of response he has been getting from his parents.

Alternative behaviors   What if the doctor looks up at Miss Alys and informs her that the young man is a well-known athlete and honor student at the University to which the hospital is attached? Would she respond with incredulous disbelief? Apologetic chagrin? Or will she merely defend herself by saying, "Well, they all look like this. It's not *my* fault if he dresses like them!"

Maybe Miss Ingram just quietly challenges her by suggesting, "You don't know this patient, why do you jump to conclusions about what he's like?" Or Miss Ingram may merely shrug her shoulders and go back to work, because she agrees.

The young man may seem to confirm Miss Alys's view of him and, at the same time, show that he, too, holds stereotypes, when he says, "You solid types are all alike. You think you've got it made because you wear a uniform. Lady, you're nothing, and you don't even know it!"

It's possible that the young man and one of the other patients may make eye contact and smile, finding comfort in each other's awareness that all people are not like this. Or the other patient may reassure the young man that Miss Alys grumbles a lot, but she's got a good heart.

10. *"Marriage and career don't go together."* Two very competent nurses are being considered for the job of supervisor of nursing services at Metropolis Hospital. This morning, the final decision is to be made by the hospital administrators, and both nurses are expecting a summons to the chief administrator's office. At 10:00 A.M. the call comes. Miss Coburn and Mr. Prentiss are invited into the office together. The administrator, William Smith, starts out by complimenting both nurses on their top-level capabilities and their excellent records. Then he goes on to say, "Miss Coburn, there is no question about your qualifications for the job, but I am sure you understand our position. You are engaged to be married. This job needs someone who can commit himself totally. You will undoubtedly be very busy with your marriage; then you will want a family. You will not be able to give enough of your thought and energy to the job. Therefore, we have decided to offer it to Mr. Prentiss. Again, believe me, it's not because you are not completely qualified professionally."

Now what happens?

Feelings   Do you think that Miss Coburn sees the logic of the administrator's position and is quite willing to wait for marriage and children in her present position? Or does it occur to her that no one has mentioned that Mr. Prentiss, too, is engaged to be married? Why should her engagement keep her from professional advancement, whereas Mr. Prentiss's does not?

Perhaps she is so overwhelmed with feelings of frustration and powerlessness that she can hardly stand it. It seems so unfair!

Is Mr. Prentiss quite satisfied that he is obviously being given preference because he is a man? Does he see the justice of the administrator's position, or is he uncomfortable about being put in the position of having his sex take on more importance than his ability?

Does Mr. Smith's apparent complacency about his stand go deep, or is he really ambivalent about what he is doing? Has he reached this decision after consulting with women as well as men, or were those who participated in the decision-making only men?

Alternative behaviors   Miss Coburn bursts into tears and runs from the room, and the two men understand and sympathize. They tell each other so: "Poor girl. She's disappointed." And that's the way women respond to disappointment, yes? Then the administrator shakes hands with the new supervisor of nursing services, and they both get on with their respective jobs.

Or maybe Miss Coburn doesn't make it quite so easy for them. Suppose she says, "You have no right to make such a decision for me, based on your prediction of my future! I will contest this decision!"

Mr. Smith announces, "This decision is final. We have made it with the best interests of all concerned in mind." He makes it clear that the interview is at an end.

Or Mr. Smith tries to placate Miss Coburn with vague promises about considering her for future advancement.

Or Mr. Smith reacts with shock and surprise, because he never suspected that Miss Coburn—or any other woman—felt this way.

Does Mr. Prentiss take a stand? Does he say that he would like fair consideration for all applicants for the job? Does he just remain silent, embarrassed about the display of emotion? Or does he remain silent because he feels he has nothing to gain by sticking his neck out?

Perhaps a fleeting thought occurs to him. If the job is definitely his, then he will have to maintain amicable working relations with many *women*. Is the women's movement for equality something to be reckoned with within the walls of the hospital?

PRACTICING INTERACTION SKILLS

In the course of role-playing a variety of situations, you may discover that there are certain specific skills that are giving you the most trouble: dealing with a direct insult, responding to a subtle slur, taking some action when a friend or colleague is denigrated, expressing anger or other strong feeling. It may be a good idea to take some time to practice these behaviors until you feel more comfortable with them. Although role-playing does provide practice, intensive focusing on specific behaviors is sometimes needed to make role-playing more productive. That is, if a wide variety of behaviors comes more naturally to you, you will be able to use them more readily to arrive at alternative solutions in the role-playing.

For this purpose, you can try the following exercise:

Go through the sections marked *Alternative behaviors* in this chapter and list those behaviors, together with a word or two about the circumstances surrounding them. For example: (1) expressing anger when someone insults your race or religion; (2) responding calmly when someone insults your race or religion; (3) offering information to correct a racial misconception; (4) protecting someone else whose nationality group is being denigrated; (5) offering support to someone whose race is being insulted.

Pair off with another member of the class. It would be a good idea to pair off with someone of another racial, religious, nationality, or sex group than your own. People of different groups bring to any problem diverse experiences and different feelings that can contribute to understanding and the development of sensitivity.

Now, choose a behavior on your list and act it out. Take turns demonstrating the behavior, showing how you would do it differently. If there are some behaviors you have never used, because you don't like them, feel uncomfortable with them, or disapprove of them, you might like to try them in this relatively safe situation: you are with only one other person, and you are, after all, only role-playing. You may just discover that a behavior you never thought you could use makes you feel great when you engage in it. You may learn that a behavior you were afraid to use is completely accepted by another person. You may find ways of behaving you never thought of before, that open for you a whole new way of interacting.

Another approach to skill practice draws directly on the group's personal experiences with prejudice and discrimination. Everyone take a stack of cards or small sheets of paper. On each card write a statement you have heard that reveals a misconception or a stereotype about a racial, religious, nationality, sex, or age group. Or the statement may merely indicate a negative feeling about a group, or about an individual because he is a member of that group.

Some statements that groups of nurses have recorded in this way include:

> Negroes could get a job if they wanted one.
> Those Jews are really cheap.
> You people. . . .
> They wouldn't live in the ghetto if they didn't want to.
> Black to white: You'll never understand.
> All Negroes talk alike.
> I can work with all people. I know how to talk to them. They like me.
> White people have good hair.
> You don't mean you go out into this community at night?
> Redheads are hot-tempered.
> After a telephone conversation: I could tell he was Negro by his voice.
> White cracker!
> Nursing is a woman's job.

When everyone has written down all the statements, divide into groups of six or eight people and begin to examine what you have written. First, discuss each statement to explore its meaning, conjecturing about the experiences, motives, beliefs, and feelings of the person who makes such a statement and helping everyone in the group understand why such a statement hurts, angers, or annoys people.

When everyone is satisfied that the statement is understood, see if you can find some effective ways of dealing with it. For example, what can you do when the statement is directed against you and your group membership? What can you do when the statement is made to you about someone else? What can you do when you are a bystander and the statement is directed against a third party? You may—without leaving your seats—briefly role-play a variety of situations in which the statement may be made, and so practice responding until you have sufficient preparation to handle a real-life situation.

4 THE NURSE
IN THE COMMUNITY

EXERCISES IN THINKING
ABOUT THE COMMUNITY

1. One of the courses in your senior year requires that you
provide some out-patient nursing care. One day you are assigned to visit
a home in the vicinity of the hospital to change an abdominal dressing on
a patient who has recently had surgery. (The hospital is located in the
heart of a low-income Black and Puerto Rican area, and your assigned
patient is a Black woman who lives in a dilapidated apartment unit about
eight blocks away.)
Your first reaction is ——————————————————————

————————————————————————————————.

Take five minutes or so to write down your feelings at being given
such an assignment. Feel free to be completely candid, because what you
write is only for your own eyes: the instructor will not ask you to submit
your paper for perusal or grading, nor will she demand that you share
what you have written with the rest of the class.

Now, working together as a group, list on the board all the feelings
that a person might have about any prospective new experience. The
feelings might be:

pleasant anticipation
great joy
fear

65

anger

some trepidation

unfocused anxiety

curiosity

Next, as a group, try to imagine why different individuals might
have these different feelings when they are given the assignment described
above. One person might feel pleasant anticipation because at last she was
being given an opportunity to be completely on her own professionally. She
has become annoyed with always having an instructor or a graduate nurse
looking over her shoulder to make sure she wasn't inflicting some fatal
damage on the patient. Even the LPNs all seemed to know more than
she did! And now—at last!—she was to administer to a patient and write
up her report all by herself. The prospect was exciting.

Another student might feel her heart drop when she heard the
assignment. She was terrified at the thought of walking into "that" community. The crime, the hostility to whites, the junkies—she had heard
and read all about it, and she *knew* it just wasn't safe for a white person to
venture too far away from the hospital. Her family was very upset when
they heard that she had decided to go to school here. She had managed
to calm them down by assuring them that she would take no risks. Now
here was her instructor practically forcing her into such danger. She was
so frightened she could not even hear what was going on in class.

Jim was furious. What right did any instructor have to make
students leave their legitimate learning areas? They could make you come
to class and they could require you to work on the floor, but there was no
law that said they could force you to work in other people's houses! He
was not planning to be a public health nurse, nor to provide primary health
care. He was going to work in a hospital, and he saw no justification for
being compelled to undertake such an assignment. The more he thought
about it, the more indignant and angrier he got. He simply would not take
this injustice lying down! He had his rights, and he was going to protect
them!

When you have explored the possible reasons for the various
emotional reactions to the assignment, look again at what you wrote at the
beginning of the exercise—your own emotional reaction. Could you see
yourself in any of the imagined descriptions? Did you learn anything about
yourself, your motivations, the reasons for your feelings? Were you
surprised that some people seemed to think there might be reactions quite
different from your own? If you want to share any of these observations
with your classmates, perhaps you can get into more comfortable groups of
six or seven and talk with one another for a few minutes. Maybe one of

the things your small group can do is to try to identify all the reasons
why a nurse really needs such an experience in the community—as well
as all the reasons why a nurse does not need such an experience. Perhaps,
as you continue to explore this section, you may keep adding to the pros
and cons concerning community involvement—and make up your own
mind only when all the evidence is in.

2. Role-play the following situation:

Carol Smith, RN, is walking from the bus stop to the hospital four
blocks away. She is in uniform. It is 7:30 in the morning, and, except
for an occasional individual walking purposefully to a bus stop or a job,
the streets are deserted. Suddenly, a child of about six appears from nowhere. His face is dirty and his nose is running. He walks behind Carol
for a while, a hand up to his mouth. Carol looks back once and smiles
uncertainly, but continues walking. Finally, the child catches up with her
and taps here somewhere in the vicinity of the hip. She stops and looks
down at him. "Yes?" she says.

"Nurse?" he asks. "You a nurse?"

"Yes, I'm a nurse."

"My mother's sick. Can you come to my house?"

What happens now?

I have intentionally omitted any description of the neighborhood
or any details identifying the social class of the child. It would be interesting
to see how the role-playing fills in these gaps and if there are different
endings to the story depending on what kind of neighborhood this is made
out to be. The chances are that a poor neighborhood or a minority-group
neighborhood would elicit one kind of response from the nurse and a
middle-class or white neighborhood would make her act differently. She
would probably be more inclined to go with the child if he was dressed
in pajamas and pointed to a ranch-style home in a tree-shaded block.
If the child wore only torn undershorts and had come out of a dilapidated
tenement, she would probably be very reluctant to follow him inside.

This reminds me of the researches done on teacher behavior.
Much to the chagrin and surprise of most teachers, it was discovered that
when they ask children questions in the classroom, they give a good
student much more time to answer than they give a poor student, *even
though the poor student is in greater need of the time.*

Carol Smith will probably put forth all kinds of reasons for her
hesitation in responding to the poor child. It might be worthwhile to examine
these reasons in the light of prevailing stereotypes in our society and perhaps
explore alternative behaviors that will bring us more closely to our professional objectives.

3. One person should buy several copies of the local newspapers. (The rest of the class should promise not to read the newspapers that day.) Let him cut out the headlines (not the ones obviously dealing with national or international matters) and lead paragraphs of each article and every photograph (without the captions).

Distribute these headlines and pictures to the class, and have each person write down his conclusion on each item given to him:

a. Do you think this happened in a Black neighborhood or a white neighborhood? Why do you think so?

b. Do you think the individual in the story is Black or white? Why do you think so?

Would you like to know if this individual is Black or white? Why would you like to know this?

c. Is the person in the picture a criminal? a victim? someone who has done something positive or beneficial? What makes you think so?

Select a representative committee to collect all the answers to the questions and analyze them for trends. A number of such trends may become apparent. There may be a general assumption that the crimes of violence are all committed in Black (or Puerto Rican or Mexican-American) neighborhoods and that the criminals in the stories are all Black. This idea may go hand in hand with the belief that the victims in the stories are all white. The respondents may justify these assumptions by saying that most Black people are criminals or that most crimes are committed by Black people. (Both of these statements are false.)

Some respondents may be reluctant to identify the race of the criminals, saying that they have no way of knowing it. However, they may also reveal a desire to know the racial identification of each person who commits a crime. (These questions might be raised: "Why this need to identify each criminal by race? Isn't the significant fact that a crime has been committed? Is a crime committed by a Black man more reprehensible than the same crime committed by a white man? Does the Black criminal require different treatment from the white criminal? Just why *is* the race of the criminal important to the newspaper reader?")

The identification of the photographs may reveal that the Black people are more often thought to be criminals than are the white people pictured. And the whites are more often thought to be victims or pillars of the community.

If these trends are revealed in the class—or even if only a few people think along these lines—you may begin to see why students dread the thought of working in a poor minority community. They have come to *expect* certain behaviors of the people, although these expectations are not the result of accurate information or intensive personal experience.

Perhaps after you have done some of these exercises, you might do a problem census in the group with the question: "What do you want to know about race relations?" Then you can proceed to explore all the things about race you suddenly are able to talk about openly.

EXPERIENCING THE COMMUNITY

Nurses working in an urban hospital usually have come from distant geographical areas and find some difficulty in settling into life in the big city. It is not just a simple problem of pulling up stakes in a small city or a suburban or a rural area and going to a large, impersonal city. In these days of mass communication, we have the problem of dealing with mass-produced feelings, too. Even those people who have lived in another part of the city and come to the hospital in the "inner city," come with these same emotions.

Just what *are* the feelings that have spread across our country and are brought out in a rush whenever somebody mentions a large urban center? The predominant one seems to be fear. People are afraid of being "mugged," women are sure they will be raped on the street in broad daylight —or at least have their pocketbooks snatched. No car is thought to be safely locked up when parked on the street, because "if they can't break in, they'll just steal the tires and radiator." The first thing newcomers hear from people who have worked in the inner city for all of six months is the story of a friend of a friend who is suffering from terrible aftereffects of having a Black man make improper overtures to her on the street. And there we have it—the nub of the matter. White people are afraid of Black people; and in most large cities, the inner core is populated by Black people, most of them poor.

Not only must nurses working in the inner-city hospital walk through streets where Black residents predominate, but they must interact with patients, a significant number of whom come from these same residential areas. The fears of crime and violence seem to carry over in some transposed form to induce fear of any kind of interaction, and new medical people become perturbed at the prospect of "not understanding *their* speech," grow concerned about "the kinds of illnesses *they* have," and fear that "I won't know what to say to someone who is having an illegitimate baby."

There is, of course, gross error in the data that are used to justify the fears. It is not difficult to get accurate information about the incidence and distribution of crime.[1] However, many people are so caught up in their feelings that they cannot use facts even when they are presented

[1] See, for example, Wolfgang and Cohen *Crime and Race: Conceptions and Misconceptions* (Institute of Human Relations Press, The American Jewish Committee, New York, 1970).

with them. Other kinds of experiences must be provided for them before they are ready to incorporate the factual data into their thinking processes.

I first suggested this activity to prospective teachers who were experiencing similar feelings at the prospect of working in an inner-city school of Black children. I have since encouraged student nurses to try it, with very satisfying results for us all. This is how to go about it.

Some day, when you have half an hour or so that you need not account for to your conscience or your supervisor, mark off in your mind about four square blocks in the vicinity of the hospital. Then take a leisurely stroll through the area, go into a store or two and buy a small item, nod and smile to people sitting in front of their homes and perhaps stop to say a word to one of them. If someone asks you why you are in a neighborhood where you are obviously not a resident, say honestly what you are doing. After all, you are a nurse in the local hospital, and you want a chance to get to know the people in the community where you work. You will be surprised at how willing people will be to help you feel accepted in their community and to help you learn what you need to know to make your nursing more effective.

As you walk, look not only at your physical surroundings and the people you meet, but also look within yourself and make mental note of your feelings and perceptions. For example, here you pass an alley blocked up with trash; what do you think? There a child just learning to walk clutches your skirt; how does that make you feel? An abandoned building with children playing in it makes you think of the dangers to them. A newly painted, carefully maintained home in the midst of dilapidation surprises you. You thought that the people would be hostile, but you find them friendly—or as indifferent as your own neighbors. You thought that you would be very frightened, but when some people respond to your smile, your fear vanishes. You thought the sounds and sights would be completely foreign, but when you see a shop selling pretty blouses, or a church of your own denomination, you feel more at home.

Come back from your walk and share your thoughts and feelings with colleagues who have done the same thing. Do you feel a little more comfortable about working in the community now? Do you think it may be worthwhile to get to know the people a little better? Do you even feel that there are some things about the neighborhood that actually make you feel comfortable, or give you pleasure?

COMMUNITY ACTIVITIES OF NURSES

In our approach to all kinds of problems faced by individuals, we are becoming somewhat more realistic. We are realizing that the child who is not learning to read, the mother who is on welfare, and the teenager who has two children by boys she can not identify as the fathers cannot be treated solely on an individual basis. It has become clear to most of us that individuals do not grow and develop in isolation, that their total environment must be considered and acted on if their treatment is to be effective.

It is true that no single profession—or professional—can deal with any total environment. This is a job for concerted interprofessional and governmental action. However, every single professional must at least be aware of the total life space of his client or patient, if for no other reason than that he may avoid choices of treatment that are inevitably neutralized by environmental factors.

For example, we have the old joke of the doctor who advises a long sea voyage for the sailor whose ship has recently docked in port. Or the doctor who prescribes a complete rest and freedom from worry for the widowed mother of five small children. Such prescriptions are not only useless, they increase the patient's frustration by making him believe that there is no help for him from a profession that does not appreciate the realities of his life.

Today, the nurse who tries to teach a Puerto Rican family about a balanced diet, but has never heard of plantain or thought of replacing potatoes with rice, is doomed to fail. The family will see his suggested diets as unattractive and uninteresting and will not even consider changing their way of eating. This nurse is rejecting the value of their accustomed foods, and by implication rejecting them. How much confidence can they have in him? How much can they trust him to care about their welfare?

The nurse working with people who are not of his own ethnic or social-class group might make a special point, in his initial walk around the neighborhood, to stop in at the grocery and food stores and examine the stock, buy some, and ask storekeepers and other customers how to prepare them. In the process of doing all this, he is taking another step in becoming involved in the community. People identify with him because he tells them who he is, and how he, a stranger, happens to be shopping in the store. He lets them know that he is unfamiliar with some of the foods. (By no means all of the foods are foreign to him. Most Americans eat many of the same foods, though with varying frequency. The outsider must not assume that people in a community are *unfamiliar* with certain foods; they merely choose to eat those foods they were reared on, just as the nurse eats the foods he was reared on.)

The next thing the nurse must do, if he is to help people plan their diets for optimum nutrition, is to research the nutritive values of the community foods and substitute them for the standard approved diets he has learned about in his training. Then he may try to interest three or four of the women in the community to meet with him in one of their homes and spend an afternoon experimenting with different combinations of foods. Thus, nutrition advising becomes an interesting and creative aspect of education, rather than a dull distribution of old lists that people will take politely and quietly discard as soon as the nurse is out of sight. And the nurse gains, as an incidental benefit, some appetizing additions to his own diet.

One nursing student, in her visits to patients in the community surrounding an urban hospital, became concerned at the evidence of drug addiction (including alcohol) that she saw all about her. Teenagers bought and sold drugs openly. Men and women sat on stoops, dazed, for hours. Pocketbooks were snatched every day—even in broad daylight—to pay for the increasing costs of maintaining the drug habit. This is not to suggest that all or even most of the people in the neighborhood were involved in this activity. The overwhelming majority of the people were poor, it is true. They struggled each day to survive in a world that seemed bent on destroying them. But they *were* surviving! Mothers rose each morning, dressed their children in the single presentable outfits they owned (kept carefully washed and ironed to be worn only during school hours), and sent them off to school with the profound awareness that in education lay some chance of their escaping from poverty. Fathers worked at jobs that paid less than minimum salaries or came back to the neighborhood after fruitless hours of trying to find a day's work. Youngsters, disenchanted with schools that by policy ignored their desperate needs, found their way to community centers, street academies, or hoagie shops.

All of them were aware of the constant traffic in drugs. Parents lived with the fear that their children were either hooked or in danger of falling into the addiction trap. They were desperate because they felt powerless to do anything about it, especially while the police commissioner denied almost daily that drugs were a problem in his city. They often confided in the student nurse and her accompanying instructor after they had finished the treatments they had come to administer. What could be done? Could the hospital help? Could the visiting nurses help?

In following through on her neighborhood assignment, the student spent some time in a local church that had turned over its basement to a group of young men. They had managed to furnish it with an old ping-pong table and a couple of easy chairs, and they used it as a meeting place to avoid being chased from street corners by the police.

Sally, the nurse, had discovered that the minister was a great source of information about the community. He had lived there for many years, had brought his new bride there four years ago, and their two children were growing up with the other children in the neighborhood. Naturally, he also was concerned about the non-medical use of drugs in the neighborhood and wanted desperately to do something about it.

One day the two of them were sitting in the basement room with six or seven of the young men talking about one of their members who had collapsed and died of an apparent overdose of heroin. Sally was moved to express in very emotional terms her anger and frustration at being unable to do anything about the situation. "I thought when I became a nurse that I could change things like this, cure people, prevent them from destroying themselves. But I'm watching it all happening and doing nothing about it!"

One of the young men told about a large hospital he had visited in a suburb about twenty miles from the city where they were treating people for alcohol and drug addiction with some measure of success. The hospital had just opened a walk-in clinic in a nearby city where people who wanted help could come.

The minister wondered if they could have such a clinic in their neighborhood, and all of them decided to speak to the administrators of the hospital and ask for advice and assistance. Ultimately Sally was the dynamic force in helping the minister organize the young men into a group that did get such a community clinic established. Sally still cajoles nurses and doctors she knows into spending several hours a week in the clinic for minor medical treatment and general physical examinations for the patients.

One nurse working in a comprehensive health services center was in a position to realize that the young people in the area could profit from regular seminars in health maintenance. She knew many of these youngsters and many of the adults in whom they had confidence and she thought that some of them would willingly attend such meetings if they were held in the health center. Consequently, she offered to make herself available at certain hours each week in one of the storefront "clubrooms" that the neighborhoods had opened for the youth of the area. At first she was asked an occasional question by someone who happened to be in the room with her. Eventually, however, she found that more and more people "happened" to be there during her announced hours, and the question and answer sessions became one of the highlights in youth activities in the community.

Another nurse saw an opportunity to reduce the incidence of lead poisoning in children caused by eating paint chips from the flaking walls of the old houses in which they lived. She had become friendly with a number of women who had been meeting in the elementary school to discuss weight problems, and two of their children had recently begun to exhibit symptoms of lead poisoning. The nurse proposed that they approach the Department of Health for help in developing a program for eliminating the hazard. After months of meetings, setbacks, and even a sign-carrying demonstration in front of the Department of Licensing, a plan was developed to use city employees and neighborhood mothers to inspect all houses for flaking paint and give notice to landlords to have the walls scraped down. In two years, only 2 per cent of the violations were still unrectified, and court cases were pending on those to make the owners comply.

A nursing student offered to take a child to the eye clinic because her mother was sick and distraught at having to care for two other children; another student offered her services to the hospital to help train a group of Youth Corps workers to be useful in the hospital setting; a RN volunteered to teach new and prospective teenage mothers attending an alternate school how to care for themselves and their babies. All these are examples of nurses who have become involved in their hospital communities in productive and satisfying ways. They did not present themselves as great change agents, out to save the benighted poor or to tell people how they ought to live. They, rather, became so much a part of the people in the community where they worked that they were able to respond to the *expressed* needs of the people who recognized their special skills and asked for their help.

Too often, people who live in communities identified as "poverty" or "minority" are besieged by outsiders who "know" exactly what they need, exactly how they must change in order to improve their communities and their lives. Millions of dollars have been poured into programs to fight the "war on poverty," yet poverty is more widespread today than it has ever been. The sad part is that if these millions had simply been distributed to the poor, they would no longer be poor!

Instead, the millions were usually given to the experts, a group characterized by great mobility. They move from program to program, from government agency to government agency, writing their reports about how the money was spent and what the estimated effects were. But the poor stay put—static and increasingly disillusioned, exploding periodically into the fury and hysteria born of unbearable frustration at having to live in a society that flaunts its great wealth in their faces while their children suffer from malnutrition.

Those experts who have begun to listen to the voices of the poor are beginning to realize that the people know exactly what they need— and by and large they know when to ask for expert help. The experts need only to make themselves available, to respond to the requests, and to refrain from assuming that they are qualified to be the prime shakers and movers.

RELATING THE COMMUNITY EXPERIENCE
TO PROFESSIONAL EFFECTIVENESS

How do you think experiences in the community can help make you a better nurse? Here is a check list of professional activities that are directly related to the nurse's community involvement. Use it to evaluate the relevance of your own professional functioning.

1. Do you feel as comfortable entering the home of a family in

the community as you do when you visit the home of a family in your own community? If people sense your discomfort in their presence, they are not likely to develop a very high level of trust in their relationship with you. If trust is a requisite in taking a nurse's advice, accepting her help, feeling hopeful when one is ill, then it is important for the patient to trust the nurse. If the nurse behaves as if she would rather be elsewhere than with the patient, the patient is likely to draw on all he knows about prejudice in our country and conclude that this nurse is just like all the "haves." She does not really care about the welfare of the have-nots, and so it is not safe to put one's self in her hands.

2. Are there many people in the community who recognize and greet you when you are on your way through it? If people know a friendly nurse in the hospital, the dread they feel about a contemplated hospital stay may be somewhat alleviated. Anyone who can alleviate some of the fears of living is to be cherished!

3. Do you see some value in encouraging out-patients to invite you to their homes for between-visit checks or just for informal visiting? The patients' home and the hospital become, then, two situational loci of the patient's total life space. Not only will both he and you feel more comfortable with each other because the division between both your fields of operation becomes blurred, but he will inevitably accept more readily your treatment and advice if you are constantly in the vicinity and available. And you will more readily accept from him corrections about your stereotypic thinking that you brought to your first encounter.

4. Do you find it almost impossible to communicate with the people in the community because you don't understand their language and they don't seem to understand yours? Often, this inability to understand one another is more the result of *expecting* not to understand than really not having enough knowledge of the other person's language. When we expect not to understand, we become so anxious that the words of the other person really do not make any sense at all. If we go into another community and speak to people, even if there is an occasional word they use that we do not know, we need only ask, "What do you mean?" to get clarification. But we feel comfortable enough to do this only if we are already communicating with some success.

5. When you are trying to help people from the community to change an unhealthy practice or institute a new health practice, do you use illustrative examples that they can relate to? For example, if you are saying that low-protein diets can interfere with growth in children and general health in adults, are you able to point out that the ground beef in the local supermarket is almost 50 per cent fat, and that you are able to tell this just from seeing the color of the meat? This is the kind of illustration that the women in the community can really learn from. They

shop in the supermarket, they buy the ground beef regularly and often, and they recognize a description of the color when they hear it. There is no point, for example, in describing what a good steak looks like when the people of this community never see one or in urging that they buy yogurt for their protein needs when they never have bought and probably never will buy this food.

     6. Do you find it necessary to maintain a non-smiling, aloof demeanor in order to get the professional respect you feel you are entitled to? It is not unusual for professional people to feel so wary of those they are working with that they are forever fearful that their status and expertise will be questioned. They are sure that if others are able to see them as the real human beings they are, then those others will not accept their professional ministrations. These professionals fear that a question about what they are doing is, in reality, a doubt cast on their professional integrity, so they comport themselves in such a way that few would dare to ask them questions. Whether it is patients or people supervised, the "professional" demeanor implies "Keep your distance" and "Familiarity breeds contempt." When they do make a mistake, then they are inevitably severely condemned for it, for those who present themselves as super-human have no right to expect to be accepted as other fallible humans are.

     What these professionals fail to realize is that the people they hold off will not share with them feelings and other significant facts. (Feelings are facts that are part of the information about any human relationship.) The nurse, for example, who thinks that everything is running beautifully on her floor because she is firm, unsmiling, and "efficient," can be almost destroyed when she suddenly realizes that the aides and orderlies detest her and cut corners when she isn't looking, and that the patients are complaining to their doctors that they are not getting the care they are entitled to. Related to this concern with maintaining a distance from patients is the whole matter of wearing a uniform and (for the woman nurse) a cap. The uniform may merely be a convenient way to dress for the kind of work that the nurse must do, and the white is convenient for checking easily any possible deviation from the high standard of cleanliness. Of course, physicians visiting their patients do not always wear uniforms.

     Some nurses may, in addition, feel that the uniform is a convenient badge for identifying a nurse, especially in an emergency when one is needed immediately. Somehow this does not seem as valid a point as it did for old-time policemen who, before they wore uniforms, were able to disappear in the crowd whenever trouble was brewing. This justification for wearing white is particularly questionable today when so many people who perform different roles in hospitals also wear white uniforms.

     Can it be that some nurses cling to the uniform because it serves to maintain the social distance between themselves and the people they treat? Is it possible that the uniform becomes one of the instruments for fulfilling the expectation that nurses not get "emotionally involved" with their patients? Perhaps the uniform makes it easier to maintain that cool air of aloofness and clinical objectivity. Perhaps if a nurse wore a green dress she might be moved to cry more readily at the sight of another's suffering—or she might be *expected* to cry.

(Of course, the women's caps are often pretty and attractive—and there's something to be said for that as a justification for wearing a uniform.)

7. When patients make references to their own lives, are you familiar with the scenes and events they are talking about? One nurse who tried to make conversation with an old man of Italian background by sharing with him some of her bowling experiences finally gave up trying to be friendly because he did not understand at all. He kept smiling and talking about "botchy" and she could make no sense of his responses. If she had listened a little more carefully, or had taken a walk half a mile from the hospital, she might have learned of the game "bocce" that Italian men had been playing in the area for generations, a game very similar to bowling.

8. Are you able to tell patients about facilities and resources in their community that they don't know about? Often people are so tied to the one block they live on that they are unaware of the many resources available to them just a short distance away. They may not know about the settlement house that is offering advice on medicare and social security, or the family service agency that provides counseling for a whole range of family problems. The nurse who has made it part of her business to know the community and visit all the agencies is equipped to give information as it becomes necessary.

9. When a patient from the community is admitted to the hospital or comes to the health center, can you talk together about events you have shared in the community and about community people you both know? How much better it is to be admitted to a hospital, ill and anxious, and then to recognize a familiar friendly person who is prepared to make you comfortable and help make you well. "Mrs. Brown" says the nurse, "I'm so glad you made the decision to come in. I think you'll be glad you did." "Yes," answers Mrs. Brown, "Do you remember when we were having coffee that day in Mrs. Smith's house, and she told us about her sister? Well, her sister is fine now. So, with what you told me, also, I decided to have it done." Mrs. Brown is still feeling ill and she is anxious about leaving her family, but she has not left her world altogether—she feels some sense of continuity.

10. Do you really appreciate those patients whose behavior

seems to violate your own values? The nurse who can see and admire
strength in an individual, even though he obviously is not accustomed to
bathing very often; the nurse who can appreciate the warmth and love
an unmarried mother gives to her newborn child, even though she herself
believes in the sanctity of marriage; the nurse who listens to what the young
man is trying to say rather than going into emotional trauma because he
uses obscenities to say it—all of these nurses are demonstrating that they
have taken the time to know the people and so are able to go beneath their
minor differences in behavior and to see the essential humanness that
transcends social class and wealth differentials. How many young Indian
and Puerto Rican people are rejected because they have been taught that
it is disrespectful to look an adult in the eye? The nurse who feels comfortable with such a youngster, even though she herself was taught that
"shifty" eyes meant some element of dishonesty in a person, does herself
a great favor: she has permitted herself to know honest people who will
not meet her eyes!

11. Do you feel comfortable with the patients from the community
because you recognize their holidays and share their pleasure in them?
Do you know many of the families and recognize and accept some of their
unique customs? Have you shared their meals as well as given them
professional help? Do you *like* them as they like you? Nothing is more
devastating to a relationship than to be reluctant to share another's food
or to brush off a chair in his home before sitting in it. Verbal assurances of
acceptance are rejected at this incontrovertible non-verbal evidence that
there is really no acceptance at all.

12. Do you generalize about "you people" when talking to
patients from the community? A dead give-away is the "you people" form
of address, which indicates to the people addressed that the speaker feels
a world apart from them. There is an implication here that "you people"
are different from me, and also, probably, somewhat inferior. There is
also an assumption that "you people are all alike," else why talk in this
way to a whole group comprised of many different individuals?

A nurse may generalize from one person's behavior that "You
people always do this kind of thing." The nurse who knows the community
from which her patient comes will never think in these over-generalizing
terms. She *knows* that the people in the community are unique individuals,
as are the people in her own community. Just as she never says "you
people" to a member of her own groups, so she never says it to a member of
groups not her own.

5 THE NURSE AND SOCIAL CHANGE

TAKING THE LEAD

So many professional people have the idea that although their expertise is available for help in processes of social change, they really are not the ones who should take the initiative in starting such a process or in instituting a change. Teachers maintain that it is the principals and the central administration who have the responsibility for essential change. Social workers are waiting for the "system" to change. And nurses often feel that they have all they can do to keep their profession from going too far away from bedside nursing. To become really involved in re-thinking the profession's whole approach to healing is left to a handful of organization leaders. And the relationship of health care to all the social changes occurring today seems to be a concern mainly of community people who are forcing health care changes just as they are forcing other changes in society.

There is a very significant leadership role that nurses can play in the whole process of social change. They, probably more than any single group in the medical professions, combine a high level of medical knowledge with a significant awareness of the psycho-social problems associated with health care. They also have great personal skill in relating to patients and their families. Other medical groups may have more of one or another of these attributes than nurses do, perhaps, but none has all three to the same extent that nurses do.

The logical place to take the lead in initiating change is in your own area of functioning. It makes even more sense to start on your home ground. This precept is not so easily accepted as one might think. It is often so much safer to advise *other* institutions and *other* agencies how they ought to change, but usually far riskier to tell the people in our own hospital or school that the time for change has come. The tendency is often, therefore, to keep from rocking the boat at home, even while we go out to tell the neighbors how much better they could make things if they only changed their ways.

However, this risk can be minimized. One of the most satisfying techniques is to identify people who see the thing more or less the way you do. Notice that I do not say that you must identify people who are most like you, or who share your general philosophy of life. It is sufficient to find some who, for example, believe with you that to discriminate against people because of their race is undesirable. Then take the next small step and agree to eliminate evidences of such treatment wherever you have the power to do so. This can be a rather loose pact, with no overtones of signing a blood pact to succeed or die trying. The idea is to feel secure in knowing that there are colleagues who agree with you and who will side with you if anyone gets upset about one of your attempts to establish equality of treatment. It is good to get together regularly with your like-minded colleagues to share your experiences, to explore new strategies for making changes, or simply to commiserate with one another about failures or congratulate one another on your successes.

Any attempts you make to change discriminatory practices are greatly facilitated by having a clear, *written,* institutional policy. Should a question arise about what you are doing or saying, it is a source of great strength to be able to quote the official policy that clearly establishes that certain specific behaviors are not tolerated in your institution. Although a written policy does not eliminate discrimination, it is a solid base for influencing people to change their behavior. The office worker who segregates the races in assigning rooms, the supervisor who gives the least desirable jobs to non-whites, the administrator who does not promote Black people are all vulnerable. They can be told that they are violating the institution's regulations, and formal charges can be brought against them. If a group of people are committed to changing these practices, approaching the perpetrators or even charging them formally presents a minimum risk. It is not very easy to use five or six people on a floor as targets for retaliation. Any systematic attempt to do so is too easily documented and made public.

Getting the ear of a like-minded administrator is also good strategy for change. Because all of us are—at one level—committed to equality and democracy, it is not difficult to get most people to comply with a mandate that people be treated equally. Of course, it is necessary for an institution to maintain vigilance and constantly evaluate practices. As the general norm becomes one of intergroup sensitivity and equality of treatment, those "reluctant gatekeepers" who want to keep the institution running for the benefit of their own groups are socially pressured to live up to that norm.

Imagine yourself in the role of a nurse who is administering medication to a patient. The patient, Mrs. Windon, is in a two-bed room. She has just had minor surgery and expects to be in the hospital for only three or four days. At the moment she is experiencing some pain and discomfort, but she is not very disturbed because she feels the worst is over.

Mrs. Windon is about forty-five years old, a young-looking white woman of a lower middle class family. She chats rather amiably with you, occasionally pausing for a moment to wince when she feels a twinge of pain.

Suddenly, there is a knock on the door and an orderly wheels in a stretcher with another patient on it. This patient is a Black woman of about the same age as Mrs. Windon. Mrs. Windon's jaw drops open and she catches her breath sharply. "Nurse," she says, "I'd like to speak to you privately."

"Yes? What is it, Mrs. Windon? Is something wrong?"

She beckons you closer, and whispers fiercely, "What's the meaning of this? Why is that woman being brought in here?"

You are confused for a moment; you don't understand.

"What's the matter?" you ask.

"Matter? Don't pretend you don't know! You have no right to bring her in here! I know my rights!"

You draw the curtains between the beds and try to calm your patient. Now, what alternative actions are available to you?

In order to answer this question, I think you must make a decision about your role in this situation. What *is* the function of a nurse when she encounters prejudice in the professional milieu? Some nurses maintain that their primary function is to protect the patient from undue stress. They often conclude that, in this particular situation, the thing to do is to wheel the new patient out of the room immediately and find another room for her. This will calm Mrs. Windon down and restore harmony.

But what about the stress induced in the second patient, Mrs. Janis? She will know why she is being moved out. How will this make *her* feel? How will it affect her relationships with the medical personnel, especially with those who are white? Will she feel quite so confident that they will provide her with the best possible care, or will she be wary, and even hostile, and harbor grave suspicions that they do not have her best interests at heart? Especially if they must make a choice between care for her and care for any white patient. Will she fear that the white patient will be given better care regardless of how serious her own condition is?

Some nurses would make a point of speaking to the Black patient and reassuring her that acceding to the white woman's demand does not indicate agreement with her point of view. It is more a case of giving in to a mild aberration in the interest of peace and quiet. It is doubtful, however, that most people would be assured by such statements. How often have peace and harmony been maintained at the expense of victimizing Black people, Puerto Rican people, Indian people, Mexican-Americans? Those who were victimized have not shared in the peace and harmony.

There are some nurses who would dissemble in the matter, saying they had made an error in assignment, that the second bed was already reserved for another patient. No one would be fooled by this explanation. Other nurses would say that there was no other space available, so the new patient would have to stay, even if only until another bed became empty. Neither patient would be mollified by this temporizing.

There are nurses who are beginning to see their function in such situations in terms of somewhat broader objectives. They have become familiar with the strategies for social change and they see themselves taking leadership roles to effect such change. They realize that there is no way to avoid all stress over race relations even in such a limited milieu as the hospital. Whatever the alternative chosen by hospital personnel, either whites or Blacks will feel stress, and the chances are good that both groups will. They also know, from past experience in race relations, that there is surprisingly little stress when a calm, authoritative decision is made in the name of fairness and the American Creed. These nurses say to a Mrs. Windon, "The policy of this hospital is to assign patients as they come in and according to the nature of their illness, so that we may give the most efficient care to everyone. We do not separate people on the basis of race, because there is no medical justification for doing so. Now, is there anything else I can do for you?"

The chances are that Mrs. Windon will subside, Mrs. Janis will also be made comfortable, and the two, left together with their similar needs for sympathy and company, will become very friendly. They will discover that race really is irrelevant in this situation.

Thus, the nurse does not become the agent for maintaining the status quo in race relations, in the name of optimum nursing care. The precedents she draws on for making her decision are to be found in other areas of human relations, ranging all the way from employers who refused to believe the threat that white workers would quit if Black people were hired, to storekeepers who refused to believe customers who threatened to shop elsewhere if Black salespeople were hired. Neither the workers nor the customers followed through with their threats, and, after the initial outburst of anger and bluster, emotion subsided and business went on as usual.

Taking the lead need not mean assuming the stature of a Father Groppi or a Martin Luther King. It need only mean affirming a policy of non-discrimination in calm, authoritative tones and refusing to give in to a momentary expression of anger. People in all types of institutions— educational, medical, manufacturing—not infrequently project their own fears and misconceptions onto others and believe they are giving in to external pressures to maintain institutional patterns of prejudice and discrimination, when, actually, they are acting out of their own needs to maintain such patterns. It is relatively easy to take on a leadership function in effecting change once we state categorically to ourselves that we believe in a policy of integration. It helps to know that most people will go along with a policy that is firmly adhered to.

Taking the lead may, of course, often involve greater risk-taking than the simple act of affirming institutional policy. I remember an operating-room nurse who had prepared a team for assisting a local surgeon. When the surgeon entered the o.r. he saw the nurse who was to assist him. His face became flushed, he stalked out of the operating room into the anteroom, and peremptorily beckoned the nurse in charge to follow him. Once outside—but separated from the other people waiting in the o.r. only by a glass partition—the surgeon remonstrated with the nurse: "Get her out of here. I have no intention of having her assist me. Next time you assign a scrub nurse, you check with me first!"

"Do you know Miss James?" asked the charge nurse. "Have you worked with her before?"

"No, I haven't! And I won't work with her now. You're not pushing a Negro nurse off on me just because I'm not a regular member of the staff here! I won't have it!"

His voice rose until the essence of what he was saying became clear to the people watching, including Miss James, who started to move into the anteroom to tell the charge nurse that she wanted to be relieved of duty on some trumped-up excuse. She hated to see her friend and supervisor caught in such a dilemma—to submit to the surgeon and hurt her friend (as well as do violence to her own integrity as a professional and a supervisor) or to stand up to the surgeon and risk being severely reprimanded by the administration, maybe even lose her supervisory position.

But the matter was taken out of Miss James's hands. As she opened the door to the anteroom, she heard the supervisor saying, "Doctor, Miss James is one of our best o.r. nurses. She is regularly assigned here and has worked with all our surgeons. Everyone has expressed satisfaction with her competence. Now, if you want to go on with the scheduled surgery, we are all ready for you."

The surgeon looked at her for a full minute, turned on his heel, strode into the operating room, and went to work. He never referred to the incident again, although there was much admiring comment around the hospital about a supervisor who courageously had refused to retreat from her considered professional judgment.

Part of the supervisor's courage came from the fact that she had for some time been discussing the problem of discriminatory assignments with the hospital administrators and fellow supervisors. She was well aware that there are laws that prohibit discriminatory hiring practices, and she felt confident that the hospital administrators were committed to obeying both the letter and the spirit of the law. She had also heard her colleagues say publicly that they believed people should be assigned on the basis of ability and patient need, never on race (although she realized that people often made prejudicial decisions without realizing they were doing so). At any rate, she knew that as obvious a case of prejudice as this would be condemned by the others.

It would seem, in the light of the outcome of this situation, that the apparent risk was far greater than the real risk. Similar experience in schools and businesses has usually borne this out.

An Exercise in Encouraging Leadership

One thing that often deters people from taking the initiative in making a change is the belief that they are the only ones who want to make that change. Sometimes they may be aware that people in their own job category want the change, but they believe that those in other (higher) categories could not possibly want the same thing, and so they feel powerless to do anything about it.

It might be useful to check out this assumption in a relatively safe way to see if people in different job categories really do share similar desires for change. It would be interesting, too, to see if some idea you have that you think no one else could possibly have is actually shared by others.

Think about your classes, your school, your university, your hospital, and select one of the changes you would like to see happen. Pick a change that you think is prettty far out—one that no one else could possibly care about. From time to time over a period of a week, make a point of questioning a number of your colleagues about your idea. When you speak to someone, do it when no one else is around, so that the individual is not disturbed or influenced by the presence of others. Tell the person what you'd like to see changed and ask him how he feels about it. If he's doubtful, do not hesitate to try to bring him around to your point of view. Keep track of the number of people who finally agree with you that a particular change is desirable.

The next step is to follow the same procedure with people in different job categories. If you are a student nurse, approach an RN, an LPN, a physician, an administrator. (There is no harm in telling them you are carrying out a class assignment if this will make you feel more comfortable.) Again, keep track of the number of people who finally agree with you.

At the end of the week, come together with your other classmates and share what you have learned. I think, more often than not, you will have discovered that (1) Your idea of what needs changing is shared by people all around you. (2) You would never have known that you were not alone if you had not made the approach. (3) People you see as more powerful than yourself also agree with your point of view.

When you are ready to try to effect a change, just remember that you need not begin planning with a large group of people. If you take the time to identify those few who agree with you, then you have enough support for taking a second step.

PROVIDING EXPERT HELP

The push these days—especially in communities of poor people— is for self-determination and community control of facilities that have traditionally been operated by professionals. The feeling among the people is that police departments, schools, and hospitals have largely ignored their needs and have often operated to harass and destroy them. In the name of education or law and order or medical progress, their feelings have been ignored, their strengths minimized, and their bodies used for the purposes of others.

No matter how beneficent the intent, it is inevitable that any agency or institution will operate primarily to the advantage of the people who make the decisions, and only secondarily to the advantage of all the others. This sounds like a cynical judgment and unnecessarily harsh and condemnatory of many people who have devoted their lives to doing good for others. I do not mean it this way. Rather, I see the statement as a realistic description of what happens in human interaction, and not at all as a "bad" or negative evaluation of human behavior. Actually, it constitutes the essential rationale for a system of participatory democracy. If the people who are served by an agency are the ones who are also involved in the policy and decision-making of that agency, it is likely that those policies and decisions will reflect primarily their own needs and desires. There are not many people who would vote to exclude *themselves* from employment on the basis of their race, or who would demand that the police use more force on them than on people in other areas, or that the hospital should close its emergency rooms to them because of lack of funds. The more patients (and prospective patients) are represented in the decision-making process of a hospital, the more will that hospital operate to their advantage.

Looking at the nature of the professional—the expert—and how he functions, we begin to see that professional expertise alone does not guarantee effective service to the society. Let me point out some of the drawbacks inherent in relying on experts to run our agencies and institutions.

1. *The experts do not know their clients.* When I say that the people who make institutional and agency decisions make them for their own advantage, I do not mean that professionals necessarily consciously make decisions to harm their clients. The bases for their self-serving decisions are not so obvious as that. Let us take, for example, a large hospital situated in the heart of a poor Black community. The staff members often assume that they really know the people they are serving, and so are aware of what the people need. This assumption is almost always erroneous, for professionals are generally middle-class individuals whose life styles are quite different from the patients' and who have no real conception of what is going on in the lives of the people they are supposed to serve. Even those professionals who started in poverty and in neighborhoods similar to those the institution serves are usually so relieved to be out of them that their behaviors and attitudes implicitly disclaim all knowledge of them.

The medical personnel of such a hospital usually get their information about their patients from newspapers and gossip and are even afraid to walk in the streets around the hospital or enter a person's home for fear of what they will find. Almost no opportunity is taken to really get to know the people as individual human beings rather than as group stereotypes.

2. *The experts believe they are expert in fields not their own.* Experts not infrequently believe that they know what is best for their clients because they are the experts, and their clients are unschooled in making such decisions. This is a belief that is most difficult to shake. But it is analogous to a pattern we often see in our society. If a man is a famous movie star, then we ask him his opinion of national politics and expect that he has a measure of expertise in that area just because he is famous and successful in his own field. There is a sort of spread of the effect of a person's particular area of specialization to other unrelated areas.

This is especially the case with doctors, and to a lesser extent with nurses, who are often expected to have almost godlike knowledge related to our most vital concerns and our greatest anxieties. The expectation that this knowledge covers not only clinical matters but also psychological and social matters is held by the doctors and nurses themselves as well as the patients they care for. Thus, the doctor who treats a child who has fallen and hurt himself while playing on a building site may tell the mother that it is advisable to spank a child in order to teach him to stay away from unsafe areas. Although the doctor is no expert in the field of learning nor even minimally qualified in psychology, he does not hesitate to give such advice. (If the truth were known, he believes in spanking children because his father spanked him—and hasn't *he* turned out marvelously well?)

Similarly, I know the case of a very fine nurse with years of experience on the surgical floor of a hospital, who was asked by a school board to take on the responsibility for teaching sex education to the elementary school children. Her traditional lecture-cum-film approach supplied a few bits of information to the children but did nothing to help them develop honesty and sensitivity in their relationships with one another. Not only was her knowledge and skill in teaching very limited, but her attitudes about sex were out of date and she knew almost nothing about the thinking and feelings of children that age.

3. *The experts are defensive about their institutions.* Generations have grown up expecting medical personnel to be omniscient and infallible, and this expectation has made us blind to their quite normal human response to any situation. Like all of us, they function to succeed, to present themselves in a good light, to win approval and recognition, to be accepted and liked and loved. Consequently, they are understandably reluctant to make decisions that might reveal some deficiency or inadequacy in the institutions they operate. For example, if a citizens' group asks that a survey of admissions practices be made to determine whether or not people of different groups are admitted and assigned on the basis of differential criteria—and even are treated differentially on the interpersonal level—hospital personnel may resist the survey: resist, first, in defence of their administration, and, second, in fear of the possibility that unfair practices may be documented and made public. The rationalization—like the secrecy of government administrations—is that it is better to work quietly without fanfare to make the necessary changes. The interesting and inescapable fact is that changes are very slow and very rare. Generally, staffs become accustomed to the status quo and do not feel the pressure to change practices that patients may be finding onerous.

The conclusion must be that if agencies are to serve their clients in the best possible way, then the clients themselves must be participants in the decision-making process. In hospitals, the patients must be directly involved in the decisions that affect their hospital stays, just as the community in general must be similarly involved since everyone is a potential patient.

One may say that a very sick person could not care less about participating in decisions on how the hospital is to function. All he cares about is being left in peace to concentrate on the business of getting well. It might be borne in mind that this very sick patient may have unmet needs he is too sick to make known. Perhaps if patients and community are continually involved in the process of decision-making and change, then the very sick patient will reap the benefits of that participation during the time he cannot be active.

All of which reminds me of a television commercial once shown around the country. A child of about four is exhorting mothers to use a certain laundry detergent for washing diapers. "When I was a baby," he says, "I couldn't talk. I couldn't tell my mother when I felt uncomfortable. But babies do have feelings, even if they can't talk about them." Patients, too, have feelings, even if they are never given the oportunity to talk about them.

This does not mean that there is no room for the professional in the changing nature of public-serving institutions and agencies. Only fools exclude the surgeon when an appendectomy is necessary, or substitute a housewife for a nurse when medicine must be administered subcutaneously. The skilled professional is an essential part of the optimum functioning of any agency. But the professional's knowledge is only partial, and he needs the information that his clients or patients have in order to do an adequate professional job.

The major difficulty that both professionals and lay people have is in establishing communication between their two groups. This implies developing mutual trust as well as learning to appreciate their respective areas of competence. At some point in their careers, most doctors and nurses will probably be faced with the necessity of undertaking this very difficult job of working effectively with community people. They can get excellent preparation for this by participating in an active health team that is really representative of all concerned groups.

An Exercise in Refining Your Role As an Expert

During the next week, keep a record of the questions people ask you, both in the hospital and outside. Make a note also of the answers you give them. (Do not include questions asked you by RNs, physicians, or student nurses.) At the end of the week, bring the questions and answers to class.

In small groups decide (1) which of the questions might reasonably be considered to involve your area of professional competence; (2) which questions were asked of you *because you were a nurse,* but which could not reasonably be considered in your field; (3) the number of questions in the second category that you refused to answer; (4) if you functioned in a team, the kinds of people you would want on the team who could probably have provided answers to the questions outside your field. Would you need, for example, a woman who had reared three or four children? A widow who managed to feed her family on an allotment of surplus food stamps? The policeman who walked the neighborhood beat? The local bartender or barber who knew everyone in the neighborhood? A person who was fifteen or sixteen years old? Someone seventy-five years old? A surgeon? Someone addicted to heroin?

COMMUNITY CONTROL OF HEALTH FACILITIES

Not long ago, I visited a comprehensive community health center completely run by a board of directors mostly drawn from ordinary community people. They had no special training, no medical background, and often no great facility with the language. However, they were making policy decisions based on their first-hand knowledge of what they and their neighbors needed in the area of health care. Not insignificantly, they were usually astute enough to recognize when a decision had to be based on medical knowledge, knowledge of broad economic factors, or other information that they did not have; and they were not too ego-threatened or foolish to refuse to call in the help they needed. They made mistakes, certainly, but they were providing finer health care for the community than professionals had ever before provided.

An important aspect of their policy-making involved looking at programs and behavior of the staff from the point of view of the people who were served by the center—their own friends, neighbors and families. For example, when I asked the medical director of the center to permit six of my education students to work part time with the child patients who were having learning difficulties, she thought it was an excellent idea. However, she was not empowered to give permission without the approval of the lay board.

Consequently, my students and I were invited to a board meeting and very closely questioned about our motivation, objectives, and qualifications. Many of us learned something that day that we had not known before. A primary concern of these community residents was that we were just another group of outsiders with another plan to experiment on them and their children. All their lives they had experienced influxes of experts and professionals in various fields temporarily fired with new ideas or with missionary zeal. The fires inevitably died out, the experts departed, and the community was left to struggle with the same problems they had always had.

This board was adamant in their refusal to permit themselves and their neighbors to be used in this way—no matter how many experts recommended a program. Only when they were satisfied that we were ready to make a commitment to see our goals through to completion, and only when they were convinced that our work would be of immediate benefit to the children, did they give their permission to admit us. But they made it clear that what we were doing would be continually evaluated for the duration of the program.

We came away with a new respect for communities so often labeled "ghetto" or "poverty" or "inner-city," their inhabitants written off as incompetent, apathetic, and unable to assume the functions of self-determination.

Part of the nurse's participation in community-controlled health facilities may very well involve a new perception of her own image vis-à-vis patients. In one such mental health unit I was engaged in teaching a course in psychology that the patients had asked for. Although I knew the psychiatrist who was in attendance at the center for three days each week, I did not know the other members of the staff: nurses, psychiatric social workers, interns in the various professions, and aides. Each week, fifteen or twenty people—not always the same ones—would come together to discuss problems of personal adjustment in more theoretical and general terms than they did when dealing with their own illnesses. I worked with the groups for a whole month before I realized that one of the people attending my class was a staff nurse. She was dressed in street clothes, so there was no obvious way of identifying her by her uniform. Everyone in the group was on a first-name basis, as was she, so there was no way of identifying her as apart from the rest of the people by the way they addressed her. She wore no name tag, and she did not intrude into the discussions in a way that would indicate that she had any specialized knowledge of psychology.

She told me afterward that she had given up wearing the uniform because she felt that it created a barrier to free communication between her and her patients. It became clear to me as time went on that she suffered no loss of respect nor of professional effectiveness as a result of this departure from tradition. Actually, the pervasive feelings of warmth and friendliness that issued from the change seemed to add to the spirit of cooperation and optimism that help make treatment successful.

The other professionals in the center were also addressed by patients by their first names. This was symptomatic of the way the center was run while I was there. It also indicated the way it was continuing to develop—toward more and more control by the patients themselves and other members of the immediate community.

One morning I came in when the regular weekly meeting was in session. Some thirty-five people, most of them patients, were going down an agenda and dealing with a variety of matters. A patient was taken to task for not keeping treatment appointments; another patient was censured for not doing his share of the maintenance chores. But what came as a revelation to me was the way in which the meeting handled a staff physician whom they accused of not devoting a full measure of time to the physical medicine clinic. When they presented the evidence against him, he offered some reasons for not being in attendance. The people listened, accepted some of his reasons as valid and rejected others, and then proceeded to work out a solution to the problem that would be satisfactory to everyone.

All through the meeting, there was no indication that the patients were always lined up on one side of an issue and the staff on the other. Each problem was considered as a problem of the institution, and everyone had a stake in its solution.

At that time, although the center itself was run democratically, with patients and staff equally involved in the decision-making and the problem-solving, the top administration held the purse strings and maintained ultimate control over that center as well as other health facilities in the area. It was inevitable that participatory democracy should lead to the demand that all controls should be handed over to the people directly concerned with the day-to-day running of the center. They wanted to make budgetary allocations, hire and fire personnel, and institute the innovations they thought desirable. Although the staff that had been working directly with the patients saw these demands as natural developments in the process of self-determination that they had initiated, the administrators balked. They did not want to relinquish their control. Much of their reluctance revolved about the belief that "those people" needed the professionals to tell them what to do. They could not accept the idea that people had a right to have a major say in the decisions that affected their lives.

The patients and some members of the staff were moved to lock themselves into the center and refuse to permit outsiders to take over. Eventually a compromise was reached on its operation, but not without generating much antagonism that left a residue of bad feeling that still remains.

The press by communities to have a greater control over their own destinies is seen very often in university situations. Here the health facility includes not only a teaching hospital, but satellite clinics, and medical, dental, and allied professional schools. In recent years, the spreading growth of these universities into the surrounding communities has caused antagonism that is somewhat different from the usual town-and-gown hostility that we have seen in the past. Especially in the cities, the university has displaced thousands of urban residents without any apparent concern for what happens to them. It has functioned as an island in the midst of poverty, without offering much of its expertise and wealth to alleviate that poverty. And its medical (as well as other) programs have not done enough to deliver adequate health care to the people surrounding it.

Such urban communities are succeeding in forcing agreements with universities that imply university commitments to function as part of the community. New programs are developed and instituted with community participation in the planning. Community decay, often hastened by the expectation that the university will shortly take over certain areas, is prevented by careful planning to retain homes, to encourage businesses, and to provide ample parking space. Local residents are provided with jobs and career ladder opportunities. And hospital and other health services are expanded and brought into line with community needs.

Perhaps it is only in an institution that is run by their own communities can some patients get the kind of treatment that is most helpful. Take this situation, for example. A man who has for years been appreciated as a devoted family man and good neighbor finds himself in a hospital with a stab wound. He is under police guard because he is alleged to have been involved in a fight with his wife and a neighbor.

A nurse is very short and hostile with him, telling him to stop his noise when he groans and being a little too rough when she removes the blood-soaked towel he has been holding to his wound.

Another nurse—a friend of the first—whispers to her, "Hey, what's the matter with you? This guy's a patient."

The first nurse says grimly, "He doesn't deserve any consideration. He's just a criminal and he's lucky to be getting any kind of treatment at all!"

In his home community, the patient is more likely to be known. Treatment personnel are more apt to relate to him in terms of his whole life, rather than merely as a "criminal" under police guard; and his chances for optimum treatment are thus increased.

Similarly, when a community suffers daily from fear that its children are succumbing to drugs, it will treat those children who are hospitalized with love and genuine concern. On the other hand, there are many hospitals situated in the midst of such anguished communities, but isolated from them; and these hospitals do not have facilities for treating addicts, nor do they care to secure such facilities. If emergency treatment is provided, many medical people, without adequate training in drug and alcohol addiction, make no effort to hide the moral indignation and distaste with which they view addicts.

If your training provides for clinical experience in a hospital only, you may like to arrange voluntarily for some additional experience in a community health center. More and more, these centers will be the instruments for delivery of health care. Traditional hospitals operate passively, waiting for patients to seek them out. With the growing importance of preventive medicine, it is necessary to seek out patients and interact with them in their home communities. (The insufficient number of private physicians also adds to the need for easily accessible units close to home.)

An example of this seeking out of patients occurred recently in one large city. A team of family health workers (all residents of that community) were sent from a center to visit homes and take blood samples from children to test for lead-paint poisoning. If the blood showed a high percentage of lead, the children were referred back to the center for treatment. The extremely high level of enthusiastic cooperation of the neighborhood undoubtedly was related to the fact that the health workers were known by their neighbors, and the decision to make a concerted effort to eliminate the scourge of lead-paint poisoning was made by the community itself. This experience is in sharp contrast to the failures of many health teams that have gone into communities and been unable to get the people to cooperate with programs the professionals developed to treat and prevent illness. In this case, the people decided what they wanted to do to help themselves; in the other cases, outsiders decided what was "good" for the people and proceeded to do it *to* them.

During your time in the community health center, you may discover that the structural hierarchy that you saw in the hospital does not exist in the same way here. It is possible that you will see the patient assuming more importance in his home community—as a whole person rather than simply as an illness to be treated. You may, more and more, discover family treatment plans, with a stable health team assigned to provide continuity of preventive and therapeutic treatment to a whole family, rather than the hit-and-miss kind of treatment traditionally provided in hospital clinics. You may begin to realize that the primary goal in medical treatment is to help the patient maintain a satisfactory level of functioning in his own community. (When you work in a hospital, this goal is often obscured and success is measured by how well the patient does while he is in the hospital, not after he leaves it.)

During treatment, the less isolated the patient is from the mainstream of his life, the more likely he is to maintain control over the treatment facility. That is, he is able to take an active part in the decisions that affect him, because the facility and the people in it are a part of his community and he is a part of them. Those units that are not yet community controlled are artificially maintained as traditional treatment centers and are controlled by professionals rather than by the people who use the centers. The traditional structure simply does not fit the new location or the new objectives of self-determination and community control currently being defined by poor communities. That traditional structure is bound to be modified. If you are working in it, you can be a part of the modification process, and you may learn the new skills and develop the new attitudes gradually rather than face the shock of finding yourself forced to change all at once when a community decides it has had enough of outside control.

REBELLIONS AND RIOTS

There is something about war in a distant country that helps professionals maintain a certain perspective about their function. I cannot imagine an American nurse refusing to administer first-aid to a German in the Second World War, even though she was right in the midst of the fighting between Germans and Americans. Even in merely conjecturing about being in this situation, a nurse would almost surely say that she sees her role as a helping, healing one, and that ideology and governments are not significant when a nurse sees someone who needs the help she is equipped to give. We even have international treaties and conventions that are designed to guarantee safety and health care to wounded enemy soldiers and prisoners. (That is, if we do not succeed in killing them first.)

However, when faced with the reality of rebellions and riots in their own country—in other words, a condition of *internal* welfare—many nurses are concerned about how to define their role. Does one take ideological sides first, and then go to work only for his own side, refusing to treat the fallen on the other? Do we maintain that rioters are criminals, and so must we wait until government agencies round them up so that we can treat them under the respectable aegis of established authority?

This is not so easy a position to take in domestic strife. The sides are never so clearly drawn. The bystander is as likely to be felled by a police bullet as is the rioter. The man throwing a stone may be the father of four who has been looking for work for a whole year. The woman fighting a policeman may be a school-community coordinator who is trying to prevent the arrest of her teen-age son.

Another factor adding to the confusion of unplanned war is that the facilities for treatment are not to be found in logically strategic locations. A hospital may be in the very center of a rebellion area, and yet be administratively committed to seeing the rebels as criminals. Does this mean that the hospital will not assign personnel to go into the street and give medical aid to the rebels? Does this mean that the nurse must share the commitment of her hospital, or can she go among the rebels and treat them without fear of reprisals from either hospital administrator or government officials?

Unfortunately, such questions are not being discussed within the medical professions. Student nurses express concern while they are in training, but the graduate nurse quickly becomes so institution-oriented that the original concern is apparently lost in the business of day-to-day health care delivery and in the security of being part of a stable social organization. However, unless the social trend sweeping the world is sharply reversed, there will a proliferation of riots, rebellions, demonstrations that explode, and fears and frustrations that send people hurtling through the streets in hysteria. At some point the helping professions will have to make a policy decision—to stand with traditional establishment institutions and work to maintain their aloofness from the turmoil, or to wade right in and patch the broken bodies on both sides until men come to their senses and stop killing one another.

Medical people, perhaps more than people in any other profession, are uniquely equipped to give witness to the horror and futility of wars, both domestic and foreign. In modern American society, most people have no first-hand experience with war, and so it is not difficult for them to filter all the pain and blood through the fine mesh of ideology or righteous anger. Medical personnel hear every day the cries of pain and try all their lives to stop the flow of blood. It is not easy for them to ignore the misery that human beings experience in peace time, a misery intensified a hundredfold in war.

Some of them have added to their medical function the task of making the world more aware of the effects of the systematic destruction that is war. But nurses, doctors, and other health people ought to do more reporting than they have done in the past. Perhaps, through their words, they can help others see something of what they have seen.

If, by this time in your nursing studies, you have become involved in the life of a poor community, you may understand something of the despair, frustration, and anger with which so many people live every day. You will have learned from them how government largely ignores their plight and authority uses them as targets of harassment. If you have been out there, then you know that this statement is no exaggeration. Even as I write, the legislature of my own state has gone on a long holiday without voting on the annual budget, and all those people who must feed their children on subsistence checks that are long past due must wait until the legislature resumes its deliberations. *Children are going hungry!*

It has been amply documented in other places that the police and the whole legal system do not treat poor people the same way they treat others. Over and over again I have witnessed municipal agencies refusing to enforce housing regulations against landlords and builders in low economic areas. Big businesses that have chain stores in poor neighborhoods often charge more than they do in middle-income neighborhoods. School personnel are usually hostile or apathetic. Health care delivery is generally inadequate and sometimes non-existent for poor people. And the rate of unemployment is often twice as high as it is in a total area.

The amazing thing about people is that, with all this, they manage to live their lives day by day with so few outbreaks against the established order. Many even continue to hope that conditions will improve. Some struggle to organize themselves into power groups that will have some clout in electing responsive officials.

But when the heat of the summer reduces the frustration tolerance and the crowdedness rubs nerves raw, some small incident may easily precipitate a war. If you are a part of the community when it bursts open, do you think you will be able to lock yourself in the safety of your hospital? Will the people you have just recently been consulting with suddenly become your enemies? Will you suddenly become afraid of the youngsters you have been treating and teaching?

The chances are that, as strong a champion as you are of orderly change and safety in the streets, you will be moved to help the victims of indifference and hostility.

6 EXPLORING GROUP DIFFERENCES IN DEALING WITH ILLNESS

PREJUDICE, DISCRIMINATION, AND ILLNESS

Before you read this chapter, take the following test. It is a simple test of factual information that can be readily checked in the medical literature.

1. Black people are less likely than whites to suffer from hypertension.

2. Mental breakdowns are more common in the middle and upper classes than in the lower classes.

3. The effect of alcohol on Indians and Blacks is quite different from its effect on whites.

4. If people suffer from malnutrition in the United States, it is because they are ignorant of how to plan a balanced diet.

5. Because of the prevalence of the sickle-cell disease, Black people should be medically counseled to avoid high altitudes.

6. Venereal disease is epidemic primarily among Black people.

7. The non-medical use of drugs is merely a symptom of spreading immorality among young people.

8. Suicide is largely a white middle-class phenomenon.

The pattern of prejudice and discrimination in our society has seriously interfered with optimum health care for many different groups. Often, the observations we accept as valid information do nothing but perpetuate errors. We are vulnerable to believing those errors because they somehow fit in with our expectations concerning groups.

Actually, all the statements in the test are false. Many people believe they are true because they fit in with the habit of stereotypic thinking about other groups. If you believe that Black people are apathetic, unambitious, and not very intelligent, the chances are that you thought the first statement was true.

Similarly, the misconceptions about Black people include believing that they are not susceptible to mental illness. These errors, coupled with the errors about the nature of the diseases, help to reinforce the prejudices. This leaves us with great gaps in our delivery of health care, for as a society we are likely to limit our search for sufferers to those geographical and social areas where we expect they will be found. All other sufferers remain invisible.

For years we did little about studying and treating alcoholism and drug addiction because we assumed it represented a peculiar aberration of inferior groups. Suddenly, we are forced to realize that people of all groups are susceptible to these illnesses. However, some people are still struggling to hold on to the belief that alcoholics and drug addicts come largely from minority groups. If hyptertension, addiction, and suicide are widespread among Blacks, Indians and youth, we might look to the way these groups are treated in our society, for all three entities are evidences of turning anger inward, upon one's self, rather than directing it against the real causes of that anger.

For years, Black applicants for aviation jobs were turned down because of the belief that they suffered from sickle-cell anemia. How convenient to assume that everyone in the group had the disease, just because it was known as a disease of Black people. Today, in the name of a growing fairness, the disease is getting much publicity and more money is being contributed for research and treatment. However, the error persists that most—if not all—Black Americans suffer from it. Not only is that not true, but the disease is not even limited to Black people. It is found in different parts of Europe and Africa and is related to a history of malaria in a region rather than to race. The years of practically ignoring the disease in America went by because the people in a position to do something about it were obviously not very interested in this "disease of Black people."

The whole problem of malnutrition in our affluent society is shrouded in revelation, denial, and gross error. Medical investigators publish accounts of widespread malnutrition; legislators deny that it results from deprivation; and many public health workers are convinced that it is all just a matter of re-educating people to select proper diets. But the evidence is growing, as unemployment spreads, that there are thousands of people who simply do not have the income necessary to provide themselves with a balanced diet.

As for venereal disease, it is epidemic among young people—and that includes young white people. It is not likely that the whites are contracting it from intercourse with Blacks!

Although we are gradually becoming aware of how our group prejudices interfere with adequate health care delivery, there is one area of discrimination that is still largely ignored. The medical treatment given to prison inmates is, at best, inadequate, and more often almost primitive. As a society we make no bones about our conviction that prison is for suffering. Consequently, our financial provision for health care in prisons falls far short of what is needed. Even medical people, although they choose from a wide variety of jobs, do not usually consider careers as members of prison staffs.

What with the enormous rate of recidivism and the fear of crime that is growing far faster than the rate of crime itself, we will soon have to make a real commitment to rehabilitation and re-education of people who commit crimes. Since there can be no rehabilitation without humane treatment, health care needs will have to be met. Are we going to be able to overcome our prejudice against prison inmates, our hostility toward them, and our desire to injure them as they have injured others?

Recently, a colleague of mine was prevailed on to volunteer to teach reading to a group of state prison inmates. After she had been working with them for several weeks, I heard someone ask her how she felt about working with convicts, and if they were "different." "You know," she answered, "they call themselves residents up there, not convicts. And that's the way I've learned to see them—just ordinary people who interact with me pretty much the way other people do."

GROUP VALUES AND
PERSONAL ATTITUDES TOWARD ILLNESS

Take twenty minutes to complete the statement: *When I was sick I felt.* . . . See if you can find some reasons for your feelings in the fact that you are a member of certain groups: social class, nationality, race, sex, geographical region, and so on. Include in your statement some observations on the kind of treatment you prefer when you are sick.

I have tried this exercise with different groups of student and registered nurses with interesting results. One nurse's response to this was: "Because I was a nurse, all the doctors and nurses refused to treat me like a sick person. They seemed to think I wanted a running case study on myself, when all I really wanted was good care, peace and quiet." Here

is an example of medical personnel acting on the basis of a preconception.
Just because a patient was a member of a particular group—in this case a
professional group—certain of her needs were, in effect, denied fulfillment.

I cannot help remembering a personal experience of my own that
caused me considerable frustration, and finally compelled me to give up a
cherished dream. When I was twenty-five years old I finally took the step
I had wanted to take since I was six: I began to take piano lessons, after
a lifetime of delay caused first by lack of money and later by lack of time. I
made the mistake of arranging to be taught by a pianist who knew me as
a successful professional in my own field. Out of "respect" and admiration
for my accomplishments, she taught me not as if I were an ignorant and
untalented beginning student, but as if my maturity and expertise in
another field somehow gave me some specific advantage in learning to read
music. For my fourth lesson, she took out a copy of George Gershwin's
Rhapsody in Blue, played it through for me once very beautifully, and
told me to take it home and practice it. The task was impossible for me!
I struggled with an ever increasing sense of failure, and finally came to
the conclusion that I just did not have what it takes to play the piano.
That was my last attempt to learn! All I had wanted was some very
elementary instruction and what I had gotten was some unrealistic
expectations with which I could not cope. The piano teacher was blinded
to my real needs because she saw me only as a member of a particular
group.

In a much more serious vein, unrealistic expectations and precon-
ceptions can be severely wounding and destructive. A Black student nurse,
telling of her experience with hospital confinement, told how the stereotype
of Black people that white people have actually influenced the course of
her illness. Upon her admission, the immediate assumption on the part of
the admissions clerk and the medical personnel was that she was on welfare.
People took it for granted that she could not pay for her treatment, and
her awareness of their assumption was intensified by what she heard white
people saying about other Black patients. Every woman who was admitted
with an incomplete abortion was automatically believed to have had an
induced rather than a spontaneous abortion. No matter what illness a
Black person was admitted with, there was the expectation that he had, in
addition, a venereal disease. There were even nurses—registered nurses—
who talked about the danger to other patients of using the ward toilets.
The gross error in medical knowledge here was obviously reinforced and
spread by the stereotype of Black people as a group.

There was the student nurse of Italian background who, until she
learned to resist playing the stereotype, had difficulty in being like herself
when she was in the hospital. "I am Italian," she wrote, "and supposed to
be very emotional, and I am a woman and supposed to like a lot of fuss;

therefore I should like people to fuss over me. Actually, when I am really sick, I like to be left alone."

How would the first nurse feel about the prospect of being sick, do you think? Just because she is a nurse, she might actually be more apprehensive than if she were not a member of the medical profession. Perhaps she would feel the need to find a physician and a hospital where she was not known so that she could be sick without the trauma of being a consultant on her own case. But running from the people she knows would force her into a position of having to develop new relationships at a time when she was least able to do so, rather than being able to benefit from already established relationships. Thus, what advantage there might have been in knowing the environment she would be confined to was lost to her.

And the second nurse: How would her group membership affect her illness? Might she have been so reluctant to go to the hospital that she delayed past the point of safety? Might she have been so defensive, so apprehensive about how people viewed her, that she rebuffed overtures of friendship and isolated herself behind a façade of aloofness and even hostility, and so deprived herself of some of the psychological necessities of health care? It is even possible that some physical care may be omitted if a patient is unattractive enough, and this thought did occur to her. By her own admission, she was inclined to view as suspect all decisions made about her treatment. Such lack of trust can make people reciprocate with dislike and rejection, and this nurse simply did not trust the people who surrounded her.

Group membership apparently influenced many of my students' attitudes toward illness, although they often did not recognize the sources of those attitudes. Even the Catholic nun who said she preferred no "extraordinary measures" of resuscitation thought that she was just being stoic and resigned. To me she seemed to be speaking out of her belief that death is a return to God. One young woman insisted that doctors and nurses leave her free to make her own decisions: "Maybe you think you know what I should do, but I know what I *must* do. Respect this in me." And she went on to observe, "Maybe I react in such a way because I am an American and Americans are very independent people."

One woman whose place in contemporary middle-class society made her feel that her illness had "socially unacceptable connotations" was so embarrassed at being ill that she was distraught at the thought that people she knew would discover what was the matter. She even felt defensive with the medical people who were trying to help her, and it took them some time to discover why she was so difficult to treat.

One man was so depressed he didn't care what happened to him, until his minister-father came to see him. He reported: "He actually reached me from the religious angle and started bringing me back to a desire to live." This was something the doctors and nurses, with all their expertise, were unable to do. However, another patient, also depressed and giving up, was visited by a minister, and the visit depressed him even more. He himself had no religion, and he interpreted the visit as evidence that medical science had done all it could for him and had abandoned him.

One student wrote, "I think if I were severely ill I would be very frightened because I would be afraid of dying." And she added, "This attitude would be a result of my religious upbringing." I was never sure what kind of religious upbringing she had that would result in such a fear, because she never elaborated on her response. However, I can imagine that a person who believed in a literal hell and purgatory, and believed himself to be guilty of sin (however small the transgression), might be afraid of dying.

Religion influenced another kind of response to illness from one patient. She had an uncomfortable sense of being bad because she was sick. she was bedridden, unable to bathe, and forced to use bedpans. Still another punishment for wrongdoing, and she felt very frightened at the implication. In her delirium, all kinds of apocalyptic visions assailed her and increased her feeling of "badness" and fear.

Another patient felt "ugly" when she was ill, because the great value she put on cleanliness violated her feeling of not being clean when She attributed this to some vague religious teaching that sickness was a felt a great sense of shame at being ill because of "what I put my family through."

A man traced his feeling of great anger at being sick to the social-religious work ethic on which he was reared. He had to be *working*—although what he worked at was really of secondary consideration. And being deprived of the opportunity to work made him angry at himself.

To one woman, hospitals meant death. Given her life experiences, this was not surprising. She was very poor, and the people in her area simply did not go to hospitals. Of course, when they were severely ill, other agencies intervened and they were almost *forced* to go to the hospital. In most cases, the people died because of the severity of their illness and the long period of neglect that they had endured. So the only people this woman knew who went to the hospital never came out alive. Can you imagine her feelings at finding *herself* a hospital patient?

One Jewish nursing student thought of how guilty she felt at not being able to work when she was ill, and she attributed her feeling to being Jewish and a woman. "Jews," she observed, "tend to feel guilty about a lot of things. They always feel they ought to be doing more—about race relations, about poverty, about their families. No matter how much they are doing, they should do more. And women feel guilty more than men do in this society. They seem to be burdened down with worry and guilt. I'm just stuck with it, I guess."

Interestingly enough, guilt associated with illness seems widespread in our society, and people attribute it to a variety of causes—religious background, social ethic, family values, and so on. One woman who described herself as a "female member of a middle-class community," felt guilty about being sick because in her region, women were taught to help others, not to be helped or waited on.

In a completely different reaction to illness, one woman (whose illness was not very serious and did not make her feel very uncomfortable) laughed a lot and really enjoyed not having to go to work. When I questioned her, she conjectured that she probably would not find the situation so amusing if her missing work meant that she would not have enough money for rent and food. She felt that her social-economic class membership certainly influenced her attitude about illness, especially this illness at this point in time.

Even a doctor's daughter found some difficulty resulting from her unique membership in that group of special patients. On the one hand, the hospital personnel expected her to be demanding and generally bratty (doctor's kids *are* like that); and on the other hand, they expected her superior understanding of the problems involved to make her a perfect patient. She obliged them—and fulfilled all their expectations—by being irritable, picky, and demanding at first, then gradually subsiding into patience and tolerance. What stays with her yet is the annoyance and guilt she felt at being treated better than other patients on the floor because of her father.

With all this clear evidence that different people feel differently about illness, and that more often than not the differences are attributable to their membership in different social groups, one nurse still insisted that "Illness is universal. All people must feel the same way when they are ill." Of course, she believed that "the same way" that people felt was the way *she* felt, and she refused to admit that there might be a need for looking beyond herself in treating others.

A reason for her insistence became clear as time went on, and it was by no means a purely selfish or even shortsighted point of view. She had seen how patients in a large urban hospital were treated and she was appalled at the way people of different groups were treated. She saw poor people neglected and middle-class women pampered, while men were expected to "bite the bullet" and stay calm. What she wanted was for all people, regardless of their sex or economic background, to get optimum health care, and she rejected any discussion of group membership as a sound basis for medical decisions. She was fearful that, if group membership were considered, then individuals would be labeled with group characteristics, and individual needs would be ignored. What she needed to see was that her basic principle was fine; but unfortunately, because of the way we have been educated, we often use that principle destructively. We refuse to acknowledge that group membership affects our attitudes, and we fool ourselves into thinking that we treat each person as an individual. Without realizing it, our treatment of people is determined by our group membership and our preconceived notions about *their* groups. Unless we admit this fact, we are doomed to seeing one another through a haze of misconception. The quality of health care inevitably varies with the practitioner's perception of the patient's needs. If a nurse feels that men should not be pampered because they are strong and stoic in their approach to illness, then it becomes clear that optimum health care for men (according to this nurse) may easily deprive some men of the compassion, understanding, touching, and talking they need in order to get well. Similarly, pampering some women may only increase their sense of guilt and shame that stems from their religious or social values.

In the last analysis, of course, we must go along with the nurse who maintained that "Everyone's an individual; you can't treat a person on the basis of his group membership." On the other hand, we must be aware of the influence of group membership on the development of attitudes and beliefs. It's a narrow line we professionals must walk between overgeneralization at one extreme, and ignorance of groups at the other extreme. To see each patient as a unique individual, yet also as a product of his background and upbringing, sharing much with other individuals of similar background, is the ultimate basis for professional decision-making.

Of course, all the sensitivity and soundly based judgment disappears into the ether when we encounter someone who says: "When I am sick I like to be dependent, looked after and babied. This is because I am a woman and I like to be treated in a stereotypic way."

An Exercise in Developing Awareness

You should have a pretty clear idea by now of how you like to be treated when you are ill. Now take this opportunity to try to understand a patient who is being treated by you. If this simulation makes you more aware of the human tendency to project our own needs onto others, it may save you from error when you are working with a real patient.

Pair off with another member of the class. One of you (*A*) tell the other (*B*) how you like to be treated when you are ill. Pretend that *B* is ill and hospitalized. *A* assures him that he will be given the best possible care. She will give him the same kind of treatment that she likes when she is ill. Let *A* go into great detail about the treatment, describing both physical and psychological factors: touching or not touching, asking personal questions or remaining aloof, discussing the clinical details of the illness or acting vaguely reassuring, sharing personal experiences and expressing feelings or remaining impersonal and detached, and so on.

Let *B* now try to make *A* understand how he would feel if given such treatment.

When *A* seems to understand, reverse the procedure, letting *A* play the patient and *B* the nurse.

An Exercise in Clarifying Values

Here is an exercise to help you decide just where you stand on this issue of group responses to illness. Pick the point of view that is closest to what you believe, or write a point of view, or merely adapt one that suits you. The idea is to end up with a paragraph about which you can say, "This is what I believe."

Group Differences in Relation to Illness

1. People who are sick need peace and quiet and so should not have visitors or any other people around them except members of the health team.

2. Some people belonging to ethnic groups that are characterized by strong family organization need to have their families near them when they are sick in the hospital. For this reason, Jewish patients should be permitted visitors whenever they want them.

3. Italians are naturally very emotional, so when you have an Italian patient, it is better not to pay too much attention to impassioned expressions of great pain or anxiety. They are probably just exaggerations.

4. Every individual reacts to illness differently. The best thing to do is to ignore everything you've heard or read about racial, religious, nationality, sex, or age groups, and just take your clues from the patient about how he wants to be treated.

5. Often, patients are reluctant to reveal exactly how they feel about their illnesses. Using what general information we have about the expectations and responses of different groups as a point of departure, we must try to discover how each individual patient's response is similar to or different from the norms of his own group.

6. Our misconceptions about the different groups in our society can lead us into grave mistakes if we assume that the individual members of any group are alike in any way.

When you have completed this values clarification sheet (and it should be done alone, not in groups), you may get together with other members of the class to share your points of view; or you may prefer merely to keep your point of view to yourself at this time, and perhaps think about it some more before you commit yourself publicly. Whatever you decide as a group, individuals should be left free to make their own decisions about whether or not to express their opinions.

Relating Group Values to Patient Care: A Simulation

Play a game with the other members of your class. Choose someone you do not know very well, and move your chairs close together. Now, as you look at each other, jot down what you *think* you know about your partner: race, religion, national origin, sex, age, what part of the country he's from, and so on. From all this "information" try to determine how you believe he feels about being sick. Finally, describe what kind of nursing care he would prefer. After you have finished, compare notes with each other and see how close or how far off the mark you were in determining the kind of nursing care you should provide.

When I tried this technique with a group of senior nursing students, they started out by laughing at the silly suggestion that they could ever base professional judgments about nursing care on an individual's group membership. Before the exercise was over, many of them were chagrined to discover that they did this quite often. Thus, a person identified as Jewish was solicitously provided with kosher food, although he actually cared nothing about whether or not food was kosher. A Black person was teased about "soul food," to his great annoyance. A young person was "mothered," without considering the great store he set by independence. And an older woman who had had three children was assumed to have no need for privacy.

Relating Group Values to Patient Care: Reality Testing

If you want to use your clinical experience as an opportunity both for learning and for improving patient care, try this: The next time you are assigned to a patient who is not so sick that he cannot respond to such questions, ask him how he would like to be treated. But follow a specific procedure so that you get information that is usable and then, indeed, use it.

1. Decide which of the groups the patient belongs to that you want to focus on. Remember that any individual is a member of a

great many groups. Just for practice, pick one of his groups as a basis
for treating him, just to check out the accuracy of your judgment.

2. Ask him two or three questions designed to provide him with
alternatives from which he can choose. For example, if you decide
to treat him on the basis of the obvious fact that he is a teen-ager, and
knowing what you know about adolescents, give him these alternatives: "Would you like me to treat you as if I were your mother or
would you prefer that our relationship be more impersonal?"

3. For part of the duration of your assignment, treat the patient the
way he said he wanted to be treated.

4. However, be sure to watch for clues that indicate he does not,
after all, really want that kind of treatment. In the case of the teen-ager
who chose to be treated impersonally, you may, for instance, see
him try to suppress an urge to cry when he is in pain, and he might
very well appreciate a motherly shoulder to cry on.

5. About half-way through your assignment, give him another chance
to state a preference concerning treatment and change your
treatment to conform with his wishes.

Not infrequently, we respond verbally the way we think we are
expected to, but our behavior indicates that we feel quite differently.

This exercise may help you begin to develop some skills for
establishing communication with a patient, about which more in Chapter
10.

AMERICAN NORMS AND
THE TREATMENT OF ILLNESS

Although there are great individual variations in our feelings
about illness in this country, there are still some attitudes that are so
widely held that they constitute American norms, American ways of
looking at illness. We are sufficiently separated from other countries and
cultures, both psychologically and geographically, that we often think that
our way of responding to illness is somehow universal, and just "human
nature." We see as odd and unacceptable the responses of people in other
cultures, and often refuse even to consider that our ways are not consistent
with optimum health care. One practice that we have persistently resisted
is the one of permitting family members to help care for hospitalized
patients. We often associate this kind of practice with unsophisticated and
even "primitive" societies. For example, when a group of Romany people
camped on the grounds of a city hospital when one of their leaders was
ill, the local newspaper made much of such "odd" behavior. Many of us
have vague recollections of reading about jungle clinics in which people

cook for their bedridden relatives. We consider such behavior picturesque and rarely evaluate it seriously vis-à-vis optimum hospital care.

It is true that a few of our hospitals permit parents to stay with their sick children beyond official visiting hours. Generally, however, the feeling of hospital personnel is that parents and relatives are just in the way, interfere with hospital routine, and do not help the patient's recovery if they are too much in evidence. This attitude is even bolstered with "medical reasons": the patient needs rest, needs to be left alone, and so on. In our society, many families are delighted to agree with this attitude, since it fits in with their reluctance and even inability to spend time with sick relatives. However, we ought to consider that many patients—especially children— feel abandoned when the people they know leave them solely to the ministrations of strangers, and this cannot have a salutary effect on the course of their illness.

Actually, encouraging families to help care for hospitalized relatives is not limited to isolated cultures. Even in such a technologically sophisticated society as the USSR, members of families are encouraged to stay with their children who are in hospitals. They are even provided with places to sleep and with meals.[1] Perhaps this is part of a philosophy of interpersonal relationships that is quite different from our own, and that is reflected in the medical treatment provided. Carter even mentions in passing that "nurses and patients touch each other more [in the USSR] than is the practice in this country."

There are other norms, values, and practices in American society that apparently have an influence on the treatment of illness. The whole drive for achievement and success that characterizes our society makes many people extremely anxious about being ill (and so unable to function). It also leaves us with a residue of impatience and contempt for those who do not achieve. There still prevails among us a lurking suspicion that illness and pain are punishment for wrongdoing. With the great value we put on youth and beauty, the sick person is often perceived as ugly and unattractive. With our belief in punishment as a way of dealing with crime, we are reluctant to provide adequate health care for people in prisons. Because we are so concerned with behaviors we label immoral, we are not averse to withholding some of the benefits of medical science from unwed mothers, sufferers from venereal diseases, and alcoholics. And, not least, we still think that people are poverty stricken because they somehow are not doing what they should do, so that poverty becomes almost synonymous with immorality.

It is difficult to say how all of this specifically affects the work

---

[1] Frances Monet Carter, "Community Mental Health Services in the USSR," *Nursing Outlook,* Vol. 20, No. 3, March 1972, pp. 164–168.

of nurses and other medical people. Suffice it to say that all of us are affected, one way or another, by the standards of our society. Perhaps it behooves each one of us to examine these standards carefully, and just as carefully check ourselves out on where we stand as individuals and professionals. The clue, of course, lies in how each one of us feels when *we* are ill. If we see in our attitudes toward our own illnesses something of these social norms and values, then we have to ask ourselves if we have similar attitudes toward other peoples' illnesses.

Following is another values clarification exercise that you may use as a springboard for class discussion of values and attitudes or merely as an instrument for helping you continue privately to clarify your values.

On Being Sick

Below are five different points of view on being sick. Pick one of them or parts of several or write your own, but you should finally come up with a point of view that you can say is your own.

1. I hate myself when I am sick. I feel awful, I look awful, and know that everyone thinks I *am* awful.

2. Being sick isn't something you do on purpose, so I expect the people around me to sympathize and be kind because *they* may be sick one day and need *my* sympathy and care.

3. People who live right and take care of themselves don't get sick. When I'm sick I have only myself to blame.

4. Being sick is a perfect opportunity for getting out of the rat race for a while. As long as I'm not too uncomfortable, I enjoy it.

5. When I'm sick, I'm a burden on my family and friends. Whether it's bringing me meals or visting me in the hospital, I know it takes them away from things they'd rather be doing.

7 OLD AGE AND DEATH: PERSONAL, SOCIAL, AND PROFESSIONAL ATTITUDES

AMERICAN VALUES
AND ADVANCING AGE

Below are seven personal views of group psychotherapy for old people. Before you go on reading the text, pick the point of view that is your own or write a statement that represents your opinion.

1. Old people don't want to think about other people's problems. They are much more concerned with caring for themselves and worrying about their own problems, and they are not likely to avail themselves of opportunities for group therapy.

2. If old people begin to be aware of their own faults, they could be very hurt or even destroyed. Better to keep them doing things that take their minds off themselves.

3. Group psychotherapy would just serve to reinforce the negative attitudes of old people and remind them that they are old. It really is not very useful for the old.

4. There's not much point in investing time and money in long-term group psychotherapy. Old people have only a few more years to live, and they are better served by keeping them comfortable and free from pain and with their material wants provided for.

5. Group psychotherapy would provide old people with companionship and feelings of belonging. It would also keep their minds off their own ailments and keep them young in spirit.

6. People submit themselves to group therapy because they are aware

that they have problems they cannot solve alone. Old people share many problems in common, not the least of which are those caused by a society that is afraid of growing old and prefers to avoid confronting the fact of aging. In groups they may begin to deal with some of these problems in constructive ways.

7. Isolating old people in groups for problem-solving just reinforces the pattern of segregating the aged. More emphasis should be put on group psychotherapy for old people, but the groups should be made up of people of all ages. Problems of the aged are also the problems of those who are still young.

On the face of it, this seems a rather far-fetched connection—psychotherapy and old age. What is the significance of believing or not believing that old people should be given the opportunity for psychotherapy? I believe that a point of view on this issue indicates some general attitudes about aging and the aged.

We know that psychotherapy takes a long time and is expensive. If we feel that old people are finished and are only waiting to die, then obviously we can see no point in spending professional time and money on them. After all, what is to be gained? They're going to die soon, anyhow. How horrible this sentiment is when it is put into words! Yet our actions really say this all the time. Homes for the aged have usually been places of waiting, dull idle places where people are isolated from the mainstream of life. They seem to exemplify the sentiment that old people need no more than shelter, food, and medical care. What more do they have a right to when they have ceased to be productive?

Rejecting psychotherapy as useful for old people indicates a lack of awareness of the problems that old people have *as a group* in our society. As a group they are being forced into idleness; they find themselves isolated from other age groups; they are stereotyped as garrulous, decrepit, rigid, and having nothing to offer toward the solutions of current problems.

Generally, the feeling seems to be that the very nature of the old, and the aging process, are at the root of these practices. It is the familiar rationalization of blaming the victims for the discrimination that society visits on them. A little closer look at what we are doing quickly reveals the errors. If, as people age, they become less able to expend physical energy, then this becomes the basis for refusing to let them continue to work. However, there are many people who, although they are sixty-five, seventy, and seventy-five years old, still command sufficient physical stamina to do the job they have been doing all their lives. As a matter of fact, after they are forced to "retire" from their life's work, they are urged to do other kinds of things—like babysitting, for example—which I think takes more physical stamina than running an electric sewing machine, selling shirts, doing general office work, or private-duty nursing. Many old people find it tiring to work forty hours a week, but they could continue working for years if they could cut down to thirty or twenty hours. But as a society, we refuse to consider shorter working days for people who need them, as if there were something sacred about the hours nine to five. (We take the same stand with mothers who want to work.) We find it much easier to mark off whole groups of people and relegate them to a social tributary instead of keeping them in the mainstream of life.

The whole business of putting old people away into homes for the aged, or into "Golden Age" hotels and housing developments, is overlaid with complacency, as if we are doing the right thing. Isn't it lovely of us to provide places where old people can live together? Don't they prefer to be with "their own?" (This is the kind of reasoning that has perpetuated the ghetto.)

Just as with other groups that have been victimized by prejudice and discrimination, the effective push for change will come from the victims themselves. To belie our stereotype of the aged as feeble, helpless, and resistant to change, there have arisen activist groups of old people that are demanding to be heard. And, unlike children who, as a group, have been systematically disadvantaged by our legal and educational practices, the old people have voting power that politicians must reckon with. The Gray Panthers are no collection of shawl-swathed dodderers! Nor are any of the other organizations that are developing and acting on plans to improve the treatment of old people. The aged have become a part of the movement for self-determination that is sweeping the world.

But we have a long way to go before people of all ages feel that they are being afforded social and psychological equality. We must first put some pointed questions to ourselves, and set about finding honest answers. Why *do* we isolate the aged? Is it because we believe that their behavior is so different from the behaviors we see in other age groups? Perhaps if we interacted more, we would find that old people exhibit the whole range of personalities and behaviors that we find in the general population.

Do we really think they have nothing to contribute to the edification of the human race? Are we so skillful at solving our social problems and so successful in our human relationships that we can afford to reject out of hand the bits of knowledge that another generation may have gleaned just from living?

I think not. There is more to this insistence on separation than we are willing to admit.

CONTEMPLATING ONE'S OWN OLD AGE

Because I believed that last sentence, I handed out to each person in a class of fifty nursing students a sheet of paper with the following directions:

Go into a corner by yourself and think of your own old age.
Among other thoughts, write your answers to these questions:

Will you have improved in some ways? How?

Will you not be as good at some things when you are old? What things?

To what age do you want to live?

Do you expect to be discriminated against because of your age? How?

What would you like to do when you retire?

The responses I got offer a great many clues as to why our society
deals with its old people in the ways that it does. Many of the students,
in their late teen years and early twenties, became extremely annoyed and
irritably protested that they could see no point at all in sitting and thinking
about their old age: "I'll cross that bridge when I come to it." "I'm only
twenty; how can I think of my old age?" "There are too many unknowns;
I don't know what the world will be like when I'm old. Maybe I'll be hit
by a car tomorrow, or find out I have leukemia." When I asked them why
they thought I had given them such an assignment, most of them refused
even to conjecture about my reasons, an attitude that was in sharp contrast
to their previous attitudes about suggested class activities. After several
sessions devoted to dealing with problems of aging and dying patients,
some of the students were able to volunteer the information that their
initial resistance resulted from feelings of distress. They felt depressed, sad,
and frightened when faced with the inevitability of their own aging. However, even with this exercise early in the unit, when I overrode their
resistance and insisted that they do it, many of them revealed their fears
and anxieties:

"It's hard to project myself as being old," one student wrote,
"because with old age I associate death. It scares me to think that I'm going
to die some day. I want to live as long as I'm in good health. I'm frightened
of the unknown, or rather, death, so I'll try not to think about it even if
I'm not in the best of health. My basic urge is to live."

Another wrote, "I do not like to think about old age. Many times
I'll walk down the street and pass an elderly person. I think to myself,
'What will I be like when I get old? Will it be like this?' The questions
baffle and trouble me at the same time. To tell you the truth, I'm scared.
Death is really the only thing I'm frightened about. I'd rather not think
about it."

"It probably won't be a very pleasant time," one person was sure.

Another considered, "I think my old age will be a time of regret
for past mistakes and things left undone. My friends will be dying. My
body will be falling apart. My children won't want me living with them.
I will be unattractive physically. Any advice I may have to offer the young
will not be appreciated or heeded."

Over and over again, nursing students expressed fear of becoming a "burden" to others in their old age. We must conclude that they consider people who are old and ill as burdens, as "crosses" to bear, as "a third wheel" in a family. And they saw this, not only in personal and familial terms, but also in social terms. As one of them summed it up, "I see no advantage in being old in our society. There is no honor, no dignity to age. The discrimination against once 'normal' members of society, now old, is not recognized as discrimination. The only positive effect of my being old will be my own more accurate perception of discrimination and the frustrations that old people feel."

I remember a high school class in which we first learned about some societies that put their old people out to die in the wilderness and in inclement weather when they could no longer work and gather scarce food. We were horrified at the barbaric injustice of this practice—to think of parents as such a burden that they would not let them live out their lives in some small measure of comfort. I am sure that the nursing students who kept wishing they would live only so long as they were independent and able to care for themselves would be just as horrified at any suggestion that old people should be permitted to die rather than become a burden on others.

With such feelings and thoughts, is it any wonder that we feel moved to relegate old people—reminders of our own fears—to the background of our lives and to the ghettos of our society? It frightens us to see them, and this fear prevents us from seeing them clearly. With blurred vision, we reject and stigmatize the aged, and our fear is compounded because we know that we, too, will be rejected eventually.

Those people who seemed to have little or no fear of aging or dying usually got their positive attitudes from the experience of knowing one or two old people who continued to live fully and well. One student wrote, ". . . I think about my father's mother and hope that my old age will be as interesting, healthful and enjoyable as the life she seems to lead." Perhaps if we can commit ourselves to really knowing some old people, we may change our ways of interacting with them. In the process, we may be able to reduce our own fears of getting old, which, in turn, will leave us less reluctant to have old people around us, which will free us to get to know old people, . . . and so on.

Two of the interesting things that emerged from the responses to the exercise was, on the one hand, the stereotype of the aged that most of the students held, and, on the other hand, the assertion many of them made that they themselves would not fit the stereotype when they got old. Where there was an attempt to accept the infirmities of old age, there was also the unconscious denial that such infirmities need really be limiting. Thus: "My thinking process will be slower, but I'll find it easier to solve the problems of daily living." "I may find it difficult to understand the young and agree with them, but I will understand and realize that they must live out their hopes and beliefs the way they see fit." "I know I'll move slower, but I'll accept my limitations and work around them and not be a bother to anyone else." "I won't spend time talking or thinking about the normal aches and pains due to the aging process." "I realize that I will not be able to do things as fast as I do now, but I will remain active and alert. I hope forced retirement will be replaced with opportunities for counseling and other working roles, so that retirement will be an active life of working and traveling."

The inner conflict of fear and hope, over-generalization and resistance to fitting into that generalization, is nowhere more sadly apparent than in the words of one young woman:

"I don't want to become someone's burden but I know that is what will happen. I realize that there are certain things that I can control in later years, but the deterioration of body and mind is beyond my control." Then, in the very next paragraph, she goes on to say:

"I believe I will have improved by having experienced life and having accumulated the wisdom and knowledge that come from education and experience. There are many things that I will always be good at, and some things I will be better at."

OBSERVING THE
TREATMENT OF OLD PEOPLE

There are some direct and very serious professional consequences of these feelings and beliefs about aging and the aged; for no matter how objective he likes to think he is, the practitioner in any profession brings to his professional judgments all the attitudes that he has learned as a member of his society. Since his behaviors usually are a function of those attitudes, we may safely conclude that the interaction of doctors and nurses with their patients is influenced by the social learnings of all of them. One has only to make a conscious effort to examine the behaviors all around us to see our prejudices in action.

I asked the same students who had contemplated their own old age with such reluctance, distaste, and conflict to start just such an examination. I directed them to return to their assigned floors in the hospital and observe the treatment of patients who were perceived as old: Were there any differences between the way medical personnel interacted with them and the way other age groups were treated?

A week later they returned to class to share the results of their observations with one another. Not only were they startled at what they had observed, but they were actually outraged. Their essential need to respect another person's integrity made them feel ashamed for their colleagues. They had discovered that there was a strong similarity between the treatment of old people and the treatment of children. The age groups in between were treated quite differently.

Although a great deal of helpless dependency is fostered in all patients, the expectation of dependency appeared far more absolute for old people. Whereas a middle-aged person would be given the opportunity to bathe or feed himself, an old person with the same degree of physical incapacitation would be bathed and fed without being offered a choice. Thus, the expectation of dependency actually fostered dependency. Nurses unwittingly became the agents for fulfilling their own expectations, and the return of the patients to autonomy was, at the very least, delayed.

In the name of "caring," outrageous liberties were taken. Old women had their hair tied up in ribbons by doting nurses, old men were teased and cajoled as if they were children, and the epithets "mother" and "pop" were used in much the same way as small children are patted on the head—whether they like it or not. It was almost as if the nurses believed that old people were unable to respond to adult communication.

The reluctance to communicate on a basis of equality with old people is understandable in the light of a classroom activity I sometimes do with nursing students. Before we begin to discuss the treatment of the aged, I ask them to list all the characteristics of old people. (And, almost incidentally, I suggest that they put down the age at which a person is old. I have found that their idea of the onset of old age ranges all the way from fifty years (!) to ninety-seven.)

Given the characteristics most of them think old people have, it is no wonder that young people decide in advance that talking to the aged will be unrewarding. Who can appreciate the views of someone who is rigid and moralistic? Who can take pleasure in communicating with someone who is sad and "death-minded"? What's the point of trying to talk seriously to someone who is senile?

At the other extreme old people are viewed as "funny" and "sweet," and even "cute." Almost always they are lonely. Out of several hundred responses over a period of years, only one person ever included in his list of characteristics "wise." The closest any response ever came to appreciating skill and knowledge in the aged have been a few "good cooks" and "very neat housekeepers."

The interesting thing is that, although people's lists of characteristics are quite similar, it is not rare to see a statement appended that says something like, "It depends on the individual personality—" an intellectual disclaimer that seems not to interfere with the more affective belief in the accuracy of the stereotype.

In the treatment of old people, the awareness of individual

differences seems almost non-existent. Since old people find themselves so frequently in contact with medical personnel and so dependent on them for help, the medical professions must make special efforts to rid themselves of our society's prejudices. Even from the purely medical point of view, in the interest of optimum medical care, such efforts are necessary. We know, for example, that as we age we may fall seriously ill yet have only minor symptoms. Without adequate communication between patient and practitioner, these symptoms may not be brought to light, and adequate treatment never may be instituted.

Similarly, the maintenance of mental health is contingent on sustained communication. When old people are segregated, isolated, ignored, rejected and looked down on, they may very well retreat into the past or into fantasy (as might anyone accorded this kind of treatment). Because old people are hospitalized more often, medical personnel are in a strategic position to help them stay in contact with reality.

Probably the most insidious aspect of the treatment of the aged in our society is that they are not permitted to give. Just as we refuse to use their time and energy, so we also refuse their guidance, their wisdom, their knowledge, and—to the extent that we keep them separate from other age groups—their love. If the medical professions could only figure out ways of providing opportunities for giving during some of those hours spent in hospitals, in clinics, in doctor's waiting rooms, and in convalescent homes!

SHARING EXPERIENCES OF DEATH

Just as we seem determined to avoid associating with the aged and so keep at bay our fears of aging, so we bend every effort to avoid the fact that we will die. We have built into our attitudes about death a belief that talking about it is "morbid" and so undesirable. I have seen nurses recoil with distaste and even anger when a dying patient indicates a desire to speak about his impending death, almost as if he were making an obscene proposal. Perhaps the best preparation we can make for dealing adequately with dying patients is to face the fact of our own deaths.

It often seems easier to begin discussing deeply emotional subjects by sharing personal experiences that may be once or twice removed from the heart of the issue. In a small group of eight or nine people, telling such experiences becomes a tentative first step in developing mutual trust. If the feelings implicit in those stories are accepted by the others, then it may be deemed safe to express more revealing emotions.

Students are given such an opportunity for affective discussion by being presented with a question like, "What do you remember of your first experience with death?" Often, even if the most affective question is asked—"How do you feel about dying?"—people will begin the discussion by recalling early experiences with the death of a pet or a public figure.

In one such discussion, a woman of about thirty-five, who had entered the nursing program after giving birth to three children and seeing them off to school, told of her first experience with death just two months earlier. A friend had implored her to attend the funeral of her father. "It would mean so much to me to have you there," she had said.

The student had often taken a stand about funerals. She thought them barbaric and unnecessary, and she maintained that she would not ever be pressured into attending one. (She wanted her own body quietly cremated after death, with no public displays of sorrow or ostentation.) Now at the funeral of her friend's father, she was taken by surprise on entering the chapel to see him lying there in death. Suddenly she was sobbing uncontrollably.

"I still don't know what came over me," she mused. "What was I crying about? I didn't even know the man."

"Were you scared?" a very young woman asked. And then, without waiting for an answer, "I saw a cat hit by a car in front of my house. I was about five or six years old." She closed her eyes and shuddered at the memory.

The group fell silent, but there was none of the usual social discomfort of people gathered with nothing to say. Rather, everyone seemed preoccupied with something inside himself. The instructor wisely said nothing at all, and just waited. Too often, in the interest of "encouraging" discussion, a teacher or discussion leader interferes with some important things that must be permitted to occur during an affective discussion. In this discussion about death, the participants would have resented prodding or prompting from an "authority." They had some very strong feelings and they wanted time to put those feelings into words. Any additional questions or comments from the instructor would have taken the discussion in a direction that *he* felt was important. But the objective of the discussion was to give the students the opportunity to talk about what *they* felt was important. The frequent and sometimes long silences were taken up with remembering, with re-living the experiences, and with mustering the courage to reveal what perhaps had never been revealed before. Sometimes a silence was a way of expressing acceptance of someone and of what he had just said.

"When my mother died," the student's voice trembled and she did not raise her eyes to look at the others, "When she died, I couldn't go and look at her. I couldn't bear to see her without life."

"I felt the same way when my brother died. Everyone in the family was horrified when I wouldn't look at him. I . . . I still feel guilty—it's been fifteen years," he shook his head.

"You must have loved him very much."

He looked up at her, surprised. "Nobody ever thought of that—
that I loved him too much to bear seeing him dead. They thought I was
something unnatural."

"Weren't you also scared—because seeing him would remind you
that someday you would die too?"

EXPRESSING FEELINGS
ABOUT ONE'S OWN DEATH

Inevitably, the discussion comes to this. It may take more than one
session with some groups, but the fear and anxiety are there, as is the
need to share them with others. In writing and talking about old age, this
fear was sometimes expressed in passing. Here, in the intimate group,
without threat or judgmental reactions, the feelings are expressed and
compared and their causes are explored.

Following is part of a transcript of a discussion by eight nursing
students. The instructor had asked the group, "How do you feel about
dying?" and had then left them to their discussion. They sat in a small
circle in the corner of a large lecture hall, and, as the discussion progressed,
their voices became very low and they leaned forward—to hear one
another better and also, it seemed, to feel closer to one another.

Characteristically, the discussion started with a personal anecdote.
But, because these students had been engaged in some of the preceding
exercises, they moved very quickly to their deep feelings about their own
deaths.

Student #1:   I've never had anyone close to me die. I never knew my
grandparents. They died in Europe.

_____ (Long silence)

Student #2:   (Tears brimming in her eyes) My mother died in the
hospital. No one was with her . . . we never expected
it. . . . They sent a telegram. My father read it. Then
he said, "Mama is gone." And he began to cry. We all
cried. And we never talked about her again.

_____ (Silence)

Student #3:   (Looking down at her hands) It's terrifying . . . I
can't really believe it. . . .

Student #4:   To be nothing—to be empty of thinking and feeling—
I am scared!

Student #1:   What's the point of being scared? Death is just part of
living. You live and you die. Everything dies.

Student #5:   Oh, really! Just like that! You're not scared or anything. You won't mind dying at all!

Student #1:   Well, I'm not looking forward to it. (Nervous giggle) But I'm not gonna mope around about it.

Student #6:   I hate talking about this! It depresses me. I really don't see what good it does.

Student #2:   You've *got* to talk about it. You've got to say it out loud over and over again, until you believe it. I'm going to die. I'm going to die. I'm going to die.

(Everyone looks at her, startled, half-frightened, brows creased)

Student #7:   I'm going to die.

Student #3:   (She puts her head in her hands; tears fall from her eyes, although she makes no sound)

PRACTICING COMMUNICATION WITH THE DYING

Very early in every course in nurse-patient relationships, the student nurse asks, "What do you say to someone who knows he is dying?" There is no formula for answering this question, anymore than there are specific directions for communicating on any subject. But this I do know. If the communication is to have made any sense, it must have had its source in a kind of honesty. The patient must have been able to say—and really know the truth of it—that he is going to die. He must have been able to discuss with other mortals his fears, his expectations about the nature of his dying, and what he wants done with his body after death. The doctor or nurse who has evaded the fact of his own death can have nothing worth-while to say to someone who can no longer evade. Whatever he says will be a lie—a lie symbolized by excessive heartiness of manner, by empty denials and assurance, or by vague dissembling.

Unfortunately, too often, this situation does not even arise. Physicians, nurses, and family members engage in conspiracies to keep the information of his impending death from the patient. But so transparent are the evasions, so obviously fearful are the conspirators, that the patient usually knows very well that he is dying—and often, in a curious way, he himself conspires to keep his knowledge from the others. The farce in the midst of this stupidity sometimes involves the medical student. He finds himself alone with the patient for periods of time, and without instructions about what to say. The patient begins to talk about dying, to ask questions, to wait for answers. The student's horrified and embarrassed stuttering may confuse the patient, anger him, make him shout with frustration or hide in a shell of apathy. And the student learns his lesson well. Forever afterward, he runs from dying patients with feelings of impatience and even hostility.

I am not suggesting that professionals cannot communicate with dying people before they have come to terms with the fact of their own deaths. I do not even know if most of us have the time we need to come to such terms before we start out on our careers in earnest. Certainly those of us who are already professionally engaged must continue to treat patients while we work through this business of dying. But I do think that we can communicate more effectively out of the very process of struggling with ourselves. The words are said more easily, the feelings are closer to the surface, and the accumulating insights make us less afraid of putting ourselves for a moment in the dying person's shoes.

The role-playing you have tried before can be useful now for testing out some of the things you are learning about yourself. Because the primary idea of dealing with dying is to think about your own death, I have adapted the role-playing technique in the first exercise to provide for real, personal material to be used directly in the role-play situation. (Ordinarily, I do not have the role-players play themselves—at least at the outset. The "pretend" aspect of role-playing provides psychological safety so that people may practice alternative ways of dealing with problems without fear of attack for being wrong.)

You will notice that, in this exercise, you are not only put in the position of thinking about your dying, but you also have an opportunity to consider how you would want to be treated when you know you are going to die. Here you can practice talking to people around you who know your condition and also develop some skill in letting them know how their behavior is affecting you.

In this situation, as well as in each of the others, as you play the nurse, you are not only able to practice speaking and other behaviors, vis-à-vis dying patients, but you can get feedback on how your behaviors are perceived and how helpful they really are.

Situation #1

1. Imagine that you are a patient in the hospital. Yesterday your doctor told you that you have inoperable cancer. Since then, you have been _____. (Write here anything about how you would feel and what you would do in such a situation.)

It is now 2:30 in the afternoon. The early visitors are gone from the floor. Your nurse comes in to ask if you need anything.

2. Pick a partner from the class and read him what you have written.

3. Let your partner now play the part of a nurse who comes into your room. He is to interact with you in any way he thinks will be helpful. You are to respond in any way you feel moved to.

4. When the role-play is over, let your partner know how you felt about his approach to you, what he said, what he didn't say, and so on.

5. Repeat this process five or six or as many times as you wish with different partners, sometimes playing the patient and sometimes the nurse.

Situation #2

Mrs. James is suffering from a progressive, fatal disease. Her doctor has told her that she will be "fine," that there is nothing to worry about. He has told her husband what her condition really is. Now, as you are administering medication to her, Mrs. James says, "Nurse, I want you to tell me the truth. Am I going to die?"

What do you do?

Situation #3

Mr. Hoppins knows he is going to die. He is a man of fifty, big, rugged-looking. He has in the past frequently boasted that he has never been sick a day in his life. His wife and two grown children are already mourning him as if he were dead.

This day, as you are fixing his i.v. unit, he says, "Have you ever thought about dying?"

What do you do?

Situation #4

Mrs. Grayson is very worried. She keeps talking about her two small children, temporarily left with a neighbor. (She has no husband. Her relatives—none of them close—live 3,000 miles away.) She is concerned about bills she has not paid, an insurance policy she was in the process of buying when she fell ill, repairs that are being done on her house that must be checked. With all of these matters hanging fire, she has been unable to get from her doctor a final date on which she can leave the hospital.

You know that it is not likely that she will ever leave. She probably will not live out the month. Her doctor keeps putting off the decision about what to tell her.

As you pass the open door of her room, she calls to you; and as you walk to her bedside, she blurts out, "I know it's something terrible! Nobody will talk to me! What will happen to my children! I must know!"

What do you do?

Situation #5

In this exercise, give the person who is to play the patient a card containing the following directions:

> You are a patient in the hospital. You have been feeling pretty sick and you came to the hospital two days ago for diagnostic tests. The nurse comes in to give you medication and make you comfortable. Just imagine yourself a patient in this situation and play out the scene, taking your cues from the nurse.

Give the one who will play the nurse a card bearing these directions:

> You have just learned this patient is going to die shortly of leukemia. The doctor and her family have left it to you to decide whether you will tell her or not. You come to her bed to give her medication and make her comfortable for the night. You have decided to sound her out a little about her feelings and attitudes and then make your decision on the basis of what you learn. You say, "_____ _____ ."

8 THE HEALTH TEAM

A BEAUTIFUL IDEA

The idea of the health team is a beautiful one—a group of people coming together and pooling their resources for the benefit of the patient. Underlying the concept of the team approach to healing (or to teaching) is the realization that the patient is a complex interrelationship of psychic and somatic systems, and that no one person can provide for all his needs. In addition, *all* the needs of the patient must be considered in dealing with his illness, because all of his needs *affect* that illness and his subsequent cure. We no longer can be content with treating appendicitis, or ministering to a headache, no more than we can be content with teaching reading. There is a whole person surrounding that appendix, a whole person looking at that primer. And the work of professionals is to relate to that whole person.

Not only are the various areas of professional expertise represented on the team, but a variety of personalities and sensitivities are also there to complement one another's observations and to cancel out one another's blind spots and misconceptions. Thus, suppose that a physician should say, "Oh, you can't take Mrs. Amati's emotionalism too seriously. All Italians act that way." An aide can adjust this misconception with her observation, "She didn't act this way before her surgery. She was very calm, even though she acted pretty sad. I think there's something worrying her that we don't know about."

Or a young female nurse may say, "Oh, Johnny's just a fresh kid. What he needs is to be slapped down and he'll behave." A male supervisor may add his more empathic perception, "He's worried about being impotent. He's desperately trying to prove that his fears are unfounded."

The health team idea not only promises optimum health care for the patient, it also offers prime working conditions for medical personnel. On the team, no one is a "para" professional or a "sub" professional. Everyone has something important to contribute to the healing of the patient. What can be more salutary in a working situation than to be convinced that you are making a significant contribution? Problems of morale, of lying down on the job and of avoiding responsibility are inevitably reduced when people know that their work really matters.

The honesty, openness, and acceptance within the team begins to extend beyond purely medical matters to more personal concerns. Team members begin to feel free to bring to team meetings problems that, if left unsolved, contribute to ineffectiveness on the job. A supervisor who plays favorites, a physician who breaks the rules of sterility, a clique that creates disharmony with its exclusiveness and gossip, an aide who is so beset with family problems that she cannot speak civilly to anyone— these matters are also brought to the conference table and all members contribute their skills and sensitivities to solving them. For just as the patients are not solely pathological entities, so medical workers are not solely therapeutic entities. They are also "whole persons" and must be related to as such.

FACT OR FICTION?

Though everybody talks about the health team, nobody really believes it exists. At best, nurses and LPNs meet more or less regularly to discuss some of the patients who present special problems. But primarily, the meetings are for distributing assignments and reading directives from administration and supervisory staff.

I know of one new wing of a hospital where it is philosophically accepted that regular health team meetings are an important part of the health care process. When the building went up, every floor had a beautifully appointed small room set aside for such meetings—a room that was to be used for nothing else—not storage, or for hanging coats or for a nurses' lounge. Today, those rooms are still used for meetings and conferences, but the "health team" conferences are made up of only nursing personnel, and are primarily vehicles for distributing assignments.

Nursing students are quick to realize that the most difficult person to get to health team meetings is the physician. They—and graduate nurses, too—are quick to say that doctors are very busy and really cannot find the time for meetings, no matter how much they might want to attend.

I suggest that both doctors and nurses are merely avoiding the real reasons. Is it possible that, because in a team situation it must inevitably become apparent that *everyone* has an important contribution to make to the healing of the patient, the physician is fearful that his own role behavior must undergo some alteration? Perhaps he will no longer be able to demand absolute and unquestioning acceptance of his decisions. Perhaps he will be compelled to submit his behavior and judgments to the critical appraisal of the rest of the team. This may be a threatening prospect to a professional who has been accorded an almost revered status in our society.

And what about the nurses? Can it be that they, too, are quite satisfied to give lip service to the idea of teamwork? Is there some reluctance to face physicians across a table in an atmosphere of equality? Is it more comfortable to maintain a tacit understanding with other nurses that doctors do not know as much as they think they do? Perhaps part of the feeling of power—and comfort—lies in the realization that they are successfully fooling doctors into thinking that nurses hold them in some awe, whereas secretly nurses laugh at their foibles and pomposity. Perhaps nurses are afraid to face the fact that, as professionals, they too must insist on the freedom to make professional judgments, and that they too must assume responsibility for those judgments, responsibility that goes beyond accurately filling a doctor's orders.

I have a feeling that only LPNs, aides, and orderlies would not object too much to becoming a part of the health team. Although some of them, of course, may have similar fears about functioning as equals with the other members, most would welcome the opportunity to contribute what they know to the process of understanding and helping the patient. It would bring a new dignity to themselves and the work they do, just as it would to the doctor and the nurse. But given the attitudes toward "sub" professionals and "menial" jobs, it is perhaps less easy for them to hide from themselves their need for respect and acceptance. They cannot take refuge behind a façade of status and pretend that they are really getting the recognition to which they are entitled.

INTERPERSONNEL COMMUNICATION

There is some evidence that problems of communication among some members of the health team revolve around their perceptions of their various roles. Responsibilities of nurses and doctors are often defined in traditional terms, and it is difficult for people to alter their definitions so that they are in tune with changing expectations of role behavior. For example, many doctors feel that nurses should not take on certain medical responsibilities. They are often disturbed at the contention of nurses that their training and skills qualify them professionally to do many things that have traditionally been the doctor's job—especially when some treatment must be undertaken immediately for the patient's benefit.

Once, I asked a nursing educator why nurses do not take on the job of medical practitioner, since it seems redundant to train a whole new group of people to take on the work included in this new role. Her answer was that nurses do not want this job, because it means being under the immediate supervision and control of the physician, with no opportunity to make independent professional judgments.

There seemed to be some difficulty in merely perceiving the nursing role as an expanding one, that requires nurses to assume responsibility for broader and more comprehensive medical judgments as their area of functioning increases in scope. Rather, the medical practitioner was seen as a "sub" physician, working almost as an assistant, with little independent professional status.

How would this perception affect communication on the health team? Would the medical practitioner be expected ever to make an independent contribution, or would he merely reinforce the physician's point of view? And would the nurse feel that her medical judgment was more valid than the practitioner's? And if the nurse *were* a medical practitioner, would people feel that she was more or less qualified than a nurse to make medical judgments?

Even differences in perceptions regarding nursing qualifications may interfere with communication among nurses on a health team. There is a feeling sometimes that baccalaureate and associate-degree graduates come to the job without the necessary nursing skills. It is felt that, although they have mastered the theory and psychology of nursing, they do not have the clinical technique, and that practical nurses are more efficient than these graduates in giving bedside care. The graduate who gets this communication from those who got their training in hospital programs may become defensive, and may even counter-attack with implications that hospital programs provide low-level manual training and do not equip nurses to be truly professional. These attitudes do not encourage nurses to communicate openly with one another and to profit from one another's special knowledges and skills.

The team approach to healing depends for its effectiveness on communication. At heart it implies the right of each member to share, and it assumes that the responsibilities of sharing are fully accepted. Let us look for a moment at what goes into a team's functioning:

1. Each member of the team (whether they are working at healing or playing football) understands the team goals. Can you imagine what would happen in a football game if each of the players had different ideas about how to score a touchdown? Yet on the health team there is not always such unanimity of understanding of superordinate goals. Each member usually perceives the goal in terms of his own special skills. Thus the RN's goal is to administer medication at the right times and in the right doses. The LPN's goal is to keep the patient clean. And so on. The overall goal of achieving a certain level of homeostasis in the patient is not similarly perceived by all team members. Consequently, the second element of team functioning is not present.

2. Each member of the team understands the reason for the course of action planned in order to reach the team goals.

What often happens is that someone "in authority" usually articulates the goals of the team, and the team functioning goes on from there. The goals are rarely defined through team effort. On the team, some of the members are obviously considered takers of orders only, never givers of insights, and it is hardly ever clear to those in authority whether or not all understand either the goals or the course of action.

The inevitable cry then goes up. "Why can't they take responsibility? Why can't they follow simple instructions?" And the equally inevitable conclusions are that they are lazy, they don't care, they are badly trained. Often, however, the real reasons for the inadequate level of operation on the floor are that people have different ideas of what is important, desirable, or best. There is no common understanding that can come from thoroughly talking out a problem *from every point of view*.

3. Everyone really knows that he is on the team. How does he know? Is it that somebody has just assigned him to the team and told him to attend the meetings, or has he helped to develop the goals and had a chance to discuss, understand, and *accept* the procedures for achieving the goals? Does he really know the rules of the game? Does he know where he fits in, does he realize his own importance on the team, does he get a chance to assume responsibility, does he get appreciation for pulling his own weight? The basic rule is not competition, but complementary functioning, and it is through awareness of and acceptance of this rule that the person really feels a part of the team.

Sometimes, someone takes the ball and runs the wrong way. The function of the team then is not to ostracize, exile, or execute the wrong-way runner. First the team must close ranks and keep its losses to a minimum. Then it must take steps to prevent such an error from occurring again. The problem is to figure out how to bring the wrong-way runner back into the framework of effective team functioning. Each team member asks: How can I do a better job, and how can I help each of you to do the same?

THE OLD VERSUS THE NEW

One of the biggest problems among nurses is the constant tug-of-war between the old and the new. Nursing students first become involved in it when they are assigned to the floor as part of their training. It is implied to them in many subtle and not-so-subtle ways that what they are being taught will only have to be forgotten once they have completed their training. This is not an unusual situation in most professions, and and even in non-professional jobs. The argument is that what the books and teachers teach is "idealistic," "theoretical," and unrelated to reality; it is only on the job that the new professional learns how things *really* are, and his first step on the ladder of success is to forget what he learned in school and apply himself to *really* learning how the job must be done.

Part of this attitude stems from the need of the experienced people to assert their superiority over the newcomers. There is some feeling of threat that newcomers often inspire because they possess the potential for changing the comfortable status quo. Part of the attitude may come from the awareness of nurses who have been in the profession for some time that they have not kept abreast of innovations and so may be exposed by new nurses who have learned the new knowledge and skills. There is also the pervasive fear that the young seek only to replace the older, that the young are not interested in learning from the experiences of older people.

On their side, it must be said that younger people, although they start out in any profession awed by the superior wisdom and knowledge of their elders, soon begin to reject much of what the experienced people say and do. Partly, this is a result of their own feelings of inadequacy. The more we find fault with others, the less likely we are to be reminded of our own deficiencies. Partly, it is the result of imperfectly understanding the inter-related facets of the profession. From books and instructors and carefully selected experiences, student nurses get a picture of what it means to be a nurse. The shiny newness of the picture is misleading. It needs to be chipped and cracked and re-colored with everyday nursing practice before it begins to take on the appearance of life. Until it does, the new nurse thinks she knows exactly what her role is all about. It is only after several years that she begins to doubt that she has all the answers.

It must not be overlooked, however, that young people *do* come on the job knowing new things that are important for adequate health care. Older people do have much to learn from them, just as younger people have much to learn from the daily successes and failures of people who have been doing the job for years.

Nurses, then, from the time they are students, are drawn into this battle between the old and the new. From the beginning, when they are assigned to a floor for their one-day pre-service preparation, they are confronted with subtle implications that what they are learning will simply have to be unlearned as soon as they leave the ivory tower of "school" and come into real life. They begin to hear that some practice is good "theoretically" but that it doesn't work in the rush of daily work and the rapid turnover of assigned patients. There are raised eyebrows and snickers at suggestions and assignments from instructors who have not worked as nurses in years, and consequently teach only "from the book."

When the new graduate nurse takes her first regular job, the same attitudes prevail, only they cease to be as subtle. The new nurse is often told point-blank to forget what she learned in school. She is told that "*This* is the way we do things here," and she conforms or her working day becomes one long agitation.

Although the apparent conflict between older nurses and new ones coming on to the floor is often over the relative efficacy of different nursing methods, the real reasons for the conflict have little to do with nursing methods—or even with professional matters generally. Underlying the conflict is fear. The older nurses fear loss of status; they are afraid of being replaced by younger people; they are afraid of getting old. There is also the fear that attends their being faced with the necessity for making changes in their usual way of doing things.

The younger nurse is fearful of appearing inept, afraid of failing at a new job, afraid that her lack of experience and knowledge will lead her into serious errors. She's afraid of her new life-and-death responsibilities, and afraid that she will not be accepted by her colleagues.

So, driven by fear, both sides focus on proving that the other side's way of operating professionally is less desirable. The idea becomes not to examine a technique in terms of what it does, but to cling to it as a means of identification and self-assertion.

There is much to-do about the generation gap in our total society, and people think that the issue involves whether or not we should continue to use the same behaviors, the same problem-solving methods and the same values in living in today's world that preceding generations have used. The implication is that older people believe that the world has remained pretty much the same for generations. That isn't it at all. The fact is, we are *not* living in the same world today that our parents lived in, and many of the traditional behaviors and values simply will not work in solving today's problems. Some of the old ways still *do* work, of course, and some of the new ways are quite dysfunctional and will inevitably be discarded as their uselessness becomes apparent. I really believe that the generations in different ways and in different degrees share this awareness. The gap is a function of ineffective communication, of distance between the groups and of errors in perceiving the other group.

Take, for example, a matter that does not involve a difference in values, although it is often perceived as a clash in basic values orientation. That is the matter of using drugs like marijuana and heroin. The older generation rejects out of hand the suggestion that such drugs be made legal. They view with horror the prospect of a brain-damaged, amoral populace steeped in these drugs and taking the human race through perdition to oblivion. Yet that same older generation uses alcohol freely, even though there are scientists who have evidence that alcohol causes more physical harm than heroin does. That same older generation uses tobacco, although there is ample evidence that tobacco causes serious physical damage. (I will not even speak of the fantastic amounts of drugs used for self-dosing, many of which cause mood and personality as well as physical changes.)

It is inevitable that, when the tug of war is over, we will take a more realistic attitude toward all drugs, evaluating them in terms of their effects and really educating our children to use them only with professional advice and for medically determined needs. In the meantime, it becomes increasingly apparent that both the old and the new ways are of questionable value in improving the quality of our lives. Relating the point to nursing, when we are faced with evaluating a method of treatment, the qualities of age or novelty are irrelevant. We need, rather, to look to the objectives of the treatment and the ease and efficiency with which these objectives are achieved. Both experienced personnel and new nurses can share their expertise in this evaluation.

AUTHORITY AND THE PECKING ORDER

It has always seemed to me that the profession of nursing starts with a great advantage insofar as building the good society is concerned. The very best in nursing principles and practices rises out of the democratic concept of human relations and is consistent with it. Essentially, what nurses—as a profession—are saying is, "People matter." And this is the essential democratic idea.

"Well," someone may respond, "doesn't everybody think that people matter? That statement is rather trite and not particularly significant." Actually, a great many people—perhaps most—are not at all sure that people do matter. At best, they are somewhat ambivalent about it. World spokesmen in the same breath boast of annihilating millions and of hating war; domestic leaders declare that everyone is equal, but that some want to be equal too quickly; the man next door believes in rehabilitating criminals, but he also believes that more executions would save money and reduce the rate of recidivism.

Nurses, on the other hand, demonstrate with every step forward that they take as a profession an essential belief in the importance of people. This is not really so surprising: The main business of nursing is to improve the condition of people in direct and unmistakable ways. More and more, hospitals are becoming prototypes of democratic communities. Democracy implies that (1) people matter more than machine-like efficiency; (2) individual differences are preferable to rigid conformity; (3) no one has the right to impose his will on others just because he is rich, strong, or powerful. What also characterizes the democratic community is the on-going dynamic struggle for self-knowledge. Medical personnel, especially graduate nurses, are asking themselves, "What is my philosophy of life? How do my emotions affect my relationships with people? Are there some people I cannot accept as equals because feelings acquired in childhood still determine my behavior? How do I really feel about sick people?"

There is no real democracy and no robust mental health without self-knowledge. The democratic person and the mentally healthy person are the same, and such a person, at his work, strives to encourage the development of democratic, healthy personalities in the people around him. The profession, realizing this, is struggling to change a number of traditional practices that mitigate against democratic functioning:

1. The old external rigid discipline based on rules, regulations and reprimands is being replaced by a personal-internal, self-directed discipline that is based on an understanding of shared goals, agreement about the validity of those goals, and continuous self-examination to check and see if one's behavior is consistent with those goals. Thus, the decision to change one's behavior is a personal one, not the result of external coercion.

2. The traditional etiquette between "ranks" is disappearing. Such etiquette was not based on admiration, nor respect for greater knowledge, experience and ability. It was superficially imposed, with the result that communication among co-workers was severely limited if not cut off completely. Today, people in all treatment roles speak to one another.

A sound system of etiquette among people comes naturally out of respect for one another as people, and as individuals with unique contributions to make to mutually conceived objectives. There are those in supervision who believe the aphorism that familiarity breeds contempt. Getting to know people is not the familiarity that breeds contempt. The refusal to understand another person; the denial that he deserves appreciation; exploiting, using, and demeaning another person and robbing him of his dignity arise out of contempt for others and demonstrate and reinforce that contempt.

Although caste systems in hospitals are beginning to disappear, and the prevailing feeling may soon be more one of "We're all in this together," rather than "Who picks on whom?" there are, of course, a hundred evidences that some of the old ideas and practices die hard. At every level of operation, there are those who continue to believe that those "below" them "understand only one language." Generally, that "language" implies lack of trust, tight external control, lack of respect, and even hostility. For example, there is an assumption among some registered nurses that practical nurses need a special form of limited communication if they are to be made to do the job. The belief is that one must not explain or give much information, rather, that the LPN responds best to specific, simple directions and that it is not necessary for her to understand much about why the directions are given. Nor does she have much of value to give in the way of information. And there are still those who remain convinced that Black people do not make good supervisors or administrators; others would rather see a man in an administrator's job than a woman; and many others meekly submit to the arbitrary demands of those in authority above them—all in the name of a level of efficiency that rarely materializes.

TEAM LEADERSHIP

It seems too bad that the idea of the health team has become, in many hospitals, only team *nursing*. The *idea* is that the people in different nursing roles—LPN, aide, RN—are to meet, ostensibly to share information about the patients and decide on the most efficacious approaches to their care. However, the nursing team meeting has in actuality become something quite different.

Limited by the definition of leadership that they have learned in elementary and high school, many graduate nurses feel that an effective leader must know everything. Their conception of the leader is one who tells others what to do, checks up on whether or not they do what is required of them, and generally acts as monitor or supervisor in the working situation.

Consequently, the team meeting is rarely a team conference. It is generally merely an opportunity for the "leader" to distribute nursing assignments. The chance is thus lost for nurses to discuss patients with an eye to considering the whole person in planning his care, and making sure that staff comings and goings and other institutional discontinuities do not interfere with the continuity of patient care.

The concept of democratic leadership is still a foreign one for many people, since few of us have had an opportunity to live with it in the course of our education. Essentially, the democratic leader arises out of the group's need in a particular situation. He is not appointed by an administrator or hired because he has something called "leadership ability." Nor is he necessarily always the one who has in his background the longest period of professional education. (We all know people who are good at doing a professional job but are *terrible* in leadership positions— causing intragroup antagonisms and generally reducing the level of morale among the group members.)

The real leader on a health team may be the person—regardless of professional role—who is sensitive to the *personal* needs of the members and takes the initiative in making them feel *listened-to* and important. Such a person may say, when a speaker is interrupted, "Let's hear this. I'd like to know more about the point she's making." Here, the leader of the moment is not the physician or the head nurse who is saying, "Don't interrupt," as our elementary school teachers did. The leader is a group member who is saying to the speaker, "I think you are saying something important." And, by implication, "I think you are important." This leader also demonstrates a way of interacting in the group that encourages people to make their contributions. These are leadership skills that an aide may have, and that may be as important in the long run for the productivity of the team as the superior knowledge of surgical procedures that the physician has.

If a person has enough of such leadership skills, even if he is not the leader selected by virtue of his rank in the hierarchy, he is really the functional leader. He is the one who makes the different roles into a functioning, interacting team. Unfortunately, most of us are not ready to acknowledge such a person's leadership if he does not also have the status we accord to certain professional roles.

Perhaps real leadership should not be vested in only one person. Perhaps different members should take on the leadership role when their own particular skills are especially needed to solve a particular problem. Perhaps the problem of the moment is to help a patient come to terms with the fact of his own imminent death. It is not too far-fetched to imagine an instance in which almost every member of the team is seriously disturbed about the dying patient and makes his adjustment to him in various maladaptive ways. The RN maintains a smiling cheerfulness and is literally almost unable to hear the patient's requests for serious talk. The aide looks perpetually lugubrious, tip-toeing around the bed as if the patient had some supersensitivity to the slightest sound. It is almost funny to see his eyes soberly following the exaggeratedly careful movements of the aide, and many times I have expected such a patient to shout "boo" just to see the aide jump and run for cover. The resident surgeon is very matter-of-fact, making it clear that he does all that surgical skill can do for the patient and nothing beyond this is his concern. Only the attending physician has come to terms with his own mortality in a mature enough way so that he can provide leadership for the rest of the team in working with this patient. He has also attended a seminar on dying and has come away with some important insights that he can try to communicate to his fellow team members. The physician just naturally assumes the leadership in this situation, and everyone is grateful to have him in the group.

This does not mean, however, that a sensitive and responsive aide has no leadership function during the conferences in which death and dying are discussed. The doctor, in trying to communicate what he has learned, may not give some of the members enough time for reflection, or for putting into words what *they* feel. The aide may, with her skills, turn the focus from the doctor to another team member—perhaps just by looking expectantly at someone who appears to want to speak, or by saying, "I don't know about everybody else, but I need time to think about this."

Thus, leadership becomes a shared function, rather than only one person's responsibility. When group members all take on some of the leadership responsibility, then they also take on responsibility for the successful functioning of the group. They will not be able to blame a group's failure on the leader's failure. Nor will they be as likely—consciously or unconsciously—to cause the group to fail because of hostility to the leader.

A TEAM MEETING

The question is, then, how do we admit fears and then go on to allay them? How do we recognize our own difficulties in interaction and proceed to develop the skills we need? With self-awareness, a lessening of fear, and a repertory of skills, we may together—the old and the new, the different professions, the sexes, the races, the diverse personalities—develop a continuing process of self-evaluation with the primary objective of improved patient care. The health team offers an ideal setting for optimal interaction without fear and for the development of such an evaluation process. There are, however, certain commitments every health team member must make if the traditional conflicts are not to persist:

1. Every therapeutic technique that comes into dispute must be studied and evaluated from the point of view of its efficacy as treatment rather than from the standpoint of its identification with a person on the staff.

2. Every member of the team should be expected and encouraged to give what information he can that is relevant to the technique

being studied. Thus, in objecting to the procedure of lining people up in wheelchairs and on tables outside the X-ray room to wait their turn, the X-ray chief may insist that this provides for the most economical use of expensive equipment, without permitting the machines to remain idle while a patient is picked up from his bed and brought immediately for X-ray treatment. The nurse may protest that patients are often pulled from their rooms during visiting hours, when some of them desperately need that social time to build psychological strength for dealing with their illness. This nurse may want some veto power over the scheduling of some patients. An aide may volunteer the information that having to wait on a table in a corridor for treatment can be a troublesome experience for some patients. The feeling of vulnerability seems to be intensified, the feeling that one is exposed to the danger of needing something and not being able to get it quickly enough. Sometimes the feeling actually approaches panic. The vague embarrassment at being stared at by passersby is discomfiting. And just the dehumanizing effect of lying on a table in a corridor like something without feelings is irritating and depressing. A doctor may suggest that such feelings of panic and depression may actually interfere with a positive prognosis. Perhaps an X-ray technician may volunteer to work late at night for those patients who do not go to sleep until midnight or later, and so he provides for optimum use of the equipment during a twenty-four-hour period, even though there are time-gaps in use during the day. Perhaps an aide suggests that she will take the time to check with X-ray periodically, so that patients may be re-scheduled without having to wait in the corridors when bottlenecks occur.

Every member's input is appreciated because it is motivated by concern about the overall effectiveness of treatment—even the economic concerns are valid if they result in more money for providing patient care. Every member is listened to with interest and respect, and the team comes to a conclusion after weighing all the information.

3. The age or youth of the individual proposing the technique should be considered an irrelevant item of data.

The sex or race of the individual may be significant if they are offering data related to their own group. (The errors that groups hold about one another make this an important matter to consider.)

The professional background of the individual should be considered only as it pertains strictly to the nature of the professional training. That is, the surgeon's decision to operate must be considered only in conjunction with the information contributed by other team members. This sounds almost ridiculous in the light of how we usually function. It does not seem to make sense to say that an LPN's opinion and a surgeon's opinion should be considered as equally valid. But I am not suggesting that, when the surgeon diagnoses the need for an operation, the team should seriously consider the LPN's opinion that surgery is not advisable. However, if the LPN has learned—as the surgeon has not—that the patient's mother died while undergoing the same operation on this day exactly two years ago, she might have an important point to make about the patient's vulnerability if she were scheduled for surgery on the same day. Consequently, for this situation, the surgeon's knowledge is very important, and the LPN's knowledge is also very important.

4. Every meeting should have scheduled time devoted to pointing out the strengths of individual team members and the things they have done *right* since the last session. Especially must the team members make a point of giving such information to those people who are currently being called upon to change certain of their behaviors or give up certain accustomed ways of doing things.

Here is a transcript of a team meeting that was role-played by a group of nurses recently. They took the roles of the various medical professionals and conducted the meeting as if it were the continuation of a regular weekly health team meeting on the medical-surgical floor of a large city hospital.

Each member of the team was given a paper that read:

> You are one member of the health team on the medical-surgical floor of the hospital. The team has been meeting to discuss the patients, and in your discussion you have come to Miss Rowan. She is a woman of about 30 who has been hurt in an automobile accident. She has a badly lacerated leg as well as numerous other cuts and bruises. She must lie on her back day and night, with the head of her bed at 30 degrees and the foot at 20 degrees. She must have her leg re-dressed twice a day.
>
> She feels perfectly healthy and does not really believe it is necessary for her to lie in bed day after day for weeks—with no end in sight to this.

In addition, each person was given a clue to the role he was to play. The clue gave a partial script *of what that person was feeling or believed* about the patient, Miss Rowan.

The person playing the nurse was given a paper containing this thought about the patient:

> *Nurse* (This is your impression of Miss Rowan)
>
> She felt very uncomfortable because her hair needed washing. I offered to wash it for her, but she declined. She was very nice about it, but sort of stiff-necked—stand-offish. I guess I was a little offended.

The other team members received their appropriate clues:

Youth Corps Worker (This is your impression of Miss Rowan)

This is one cool gal. She tells it like it really is. She knows what's happening in this country, and she's not afraid to say what's wrong. I wish more adults were like her.

She feels so useless right now—she can hardly stand it.

Minister (This is your impression of Miss Rowan)

I came in to offer what comfort I could, and I couldn't get over the feeling she was laughing at me. Oh—she was polite enough, but I got that feeling.

Volunteer (This is your impression of Miss Rowan)

She borrows books regularly from my cart. She really likes to read. I tried to discuss some of the books with her, but she was very non-committal—almost as if she didn't want to talk about them. Mostly she selects mysteries and light novels.

Visiting Foreign Physician (This is your impression of Miss Rowan)

I came in to ask if I could look at her leg—I'm interested in the kind of treatment she's getting. She told me in no uncertain terms that I was welcome to see whatever I could through the bandage—and that she was not about to increase the risk of infection by letting me remove it.

Does she think she knows more about medicine than I do? As if I'd do anything to hurt a patient!

X-Ray Technician (This is your impression of Miss Rowan)

She was wheeled down to X-ray the other day to have her hand X-rayed to check for suspected fractures. She was very snippy when I told her to straighten her fingers on the X-ray plate. She said, "If I could straighten my fingers, I wouldn't need an X-ray!"

What did she expect me to do, take an X-ray improperly?

LPN (This is your impression of Miss Rowan)

She's very nice and cooperative, and tries not to be demanding. However, she almost snapped my head off at 2:00 A.M. one morning when I flashed a light to check and see that everything was all right with her—as I am instructed to do with private-room patients.

Doctor—Plastic Surgeon (This is your impression of Miss Rowan)

I come in at 6:30 in the morning and again at 6:30 in the evening to dress her leg. I have grown to appreciate her wit and intelligence, though I realize how much she wished this ordeal were over and she could get back to work.

However, she always seems cheerful and never complains.

Orderly (This is your impression of Miss Rowan)

I think she is a very educated woman and I respect her, but she doesn't speak to me as if I were beneath her. The other day I discussed the wage freeze and talked about how hard it was to raise a family on $4,000 a year.

She mentioned the other day that she hates the feeling of helplessness she gets staying in bed and having people "do things" to her. She even hates to go to the beauty parlor for this reason.

	Transcript	*Explanation*
Nurse:	I feel I know my patients pretty well, and this one is no exception. She's getting everything she needs, I assure you.	The nurse has taken the lead in the discussion: she has been "conducting" team meetings for some time. (Of course, the "teams" have always been made up exclusively of nursing personnel.) She sounds a little defensive.
Orderly:	Maybe that's what's bothering her. She's the kind of person who feels bad when people do everything for her. She likes to be independent.	
Youth Corps Worker:	Yeah—she feels so useless she can hardly stand it.	The orderly is apparently the key to her defensiveness. He has detected
Nurse:	Aren't we spending a little too much time on this patient? After all, she's hardly in critical condition! All she needs is to lie still for a few more days and she'll be out of here. (Turning to the doctor) Let's go on to some of the other patients who have some important *medical* problems, Doctor.	a flaw in her approach to this patient—and the Youth Corps Worker is corroborating it. The nurse takes refuge in underlining her superior status by allying herself with the doctor and, by implication, excluding from the conference those who are not qualified to discuss "medical problems."
Plastic Surgeon:	I wonder if Miss Rowan *could* stand some special help. I'm sometimes so preoccupied. . . .	The surgeon has some vague feeling that he is overlooking something, and
Visiting Doctor:	She doesn't want anyone's concern; a rather aggressive woman. (He shakes his head in disapproval.)	he seems receptive to additional information. Un-

	Transcript	*Explanation*

Nurse: I can understand how she feels. She's a woman accustomed to directing her own life—a successful woman in her profession—and suddenly all the control is taken away from her.

Plastic Surgeon: You know, she actually can be of help to me. I'd like her professional opinion about the interdisciplinary research we're doing on the effects of radical facial surgery on cancer patients.

Nurse: (Smiling) That should take her out of herself a little—make her feel less useless.

X-Ray Technician: (Mumbling) Hmph . . . she's above herself already.

Minister: (Half to himself) Maybe I should stop in and see her again. . . .

fortunately, the one who offers information at that moment is another physician, and the preceding more important information provided by "lower status" personnel is obscured.

The nurse rallies. She detects a note of male superiority in the visiting physician's manner, and her general sensitivity to stereotyping momentarily distracts her from ego defensiveness. She is able to get through to the surgeon.

But the X-ray technician remains disgruntled, and the minister seems to feel that his single visit to Miss Rowan was somehow inconclusive.

With an exercise such as this, a group can pick up the role-playing of this team meeting at any point. While some members play out the team roles, the rest may make notes on the pattern of interaction they observe. If one of the observers feels the need to participate at any time in the course of the role-playing, let him tap one of the team members on the shoulder and quickly exchange places with him, without interrupting the flow of the meeting.

PRACTICING COMMUNICATION "UPWARD"

Does this situation sound familiar to you? The doctor who is caring for one of your patients is simply not doing what he should. The patient has a terminal illness and is full of anxieties and questions, but the doctor either avoids coming to see him, or dashes in and out and pretends to be too busy to talk. What would you do?

Maybe the doctor really is exceedingly busy and simply cannot take any time from seeing his many other patients to sit and deal with the problems of this one person. On the other hand, maybe he is so disturbed by his feelings of powerlessness in the face of imminent death that he is compelled to run from a dying person. Perhaps he feels that he has no answers to the many questions and that he will only make things worse for the patient by admitting this. It is possible that he is unaware of the patient's questions and feels that the excellent physical care he is getting is all that need be done for him. Maybe he really is a callous s.o.b. and thinks that, since he has provided all the help that medical science can offer at this point in time, he is absolved of further responsibility, and he is free to go on to other situations in which medical science still has something to offer. Maybe he believes the nurse is quite capable of giving psychological as well as physical help without further consultation with the physician.

Whatever the attitude or feelings of this doctor may be, the nurse does not really know them without finding out what they are from him. Unless she sits down and speaks with him—perhaps at some length— she cannot learn what he thinks he is doing, why he thinks he is doing it, and what he expects other medical personnel to be doing.

But how great a risk it is for a nurse to question the behavior of an attending physician! How many nurses are prepared to do such a thing: flouting tradition, breaking protocol, acting "unprofessional"? So there is a stalemate: the patient has needs, no one is providing for them, and the professional who seems aware of them is afraid to do anything about them. The only thing the nurse can do is make the patient physically comfortable and assure him that the doctor knows just what he is doing. Right? Wrong! The nurse can learn some things about herself, her profession, and her hospital situation that will help her solve her predicament.

Here is a first step that each one of you can take. During a lull in the rush on the floor to which you are assigned, take the opportunity to speak quietly for a few minutes to one of the doctors—not an intern, not a personal friend of yours with whom you often speak, but with one of the doctors with whom you have a formally professional, no-nonsense relationship. Recount to him the situation of the "busy" doctor and the dying patient and ask him what he would want the nurse to do if he were the doctor in the case.

No matter how nervous you feel about doing this, you should know that there are several factors that contribute substantially to making this a risk-free situation: (1) There are very few people who can resist feeling good when someone asks their expert advice. One does not snap the head off of the person who makes one feel good! (2) The case is a hypothetical one and so discussing it poses no real threat to anyone. The doctor may be assured that his opinions will not be interpreted as criticism of a colleague, and the nurse need not feel as if she is complaining about someone with whom she must have an amicable working rela- tionship. (3) It is quite possible that behind that formal doctor façade there is a human being struggling with professional concerns that he would be delighted to discuss with people similarly concerned. (4) If he just wants to maintain the status quo in your relationship, the doctor is free to say that he really doesn't have the time to talk about it now— but maybe another time . . . ?

What purposes might this approach accomplish? For one thing, a nurse or prospective nurse may discover just how reluctant she is to speak with a doctor as an equal. Does this mean she feels *inferior* to doctors? Well, *do* you?

The nurse may also, faced with such an assignment, suddenly recall with great emotional force all the traditions of the profession that he has *intellectually* scoffed at and discarded: The good nurse merely follows doctors' orders without question; doctors know more than nurses do, so doctors' judgments are always more soundly based than nurses'; doctors may be rude to nurses with impunity, and nurses may not retaliate in kind. The nurse may surprise himself by realizing that, faced with these traditional precepts of his profession, he may *behave* as if he accepted their validity even though he has always *said* that they were just so much nonsense.

And the nurse may, at last, be forced to admit that no matter how progressive the hospital administrators maintain that they are, and no matter how firmly the state and national professional organizations insist that the image, the function, and the status of the nurse are changing, in this hospital professional relationships have not changed since Florence Nightingale staged a one-nurse revolution.

Now that the nurse has faced the reality of his situation in all its brutal clarity, he has some chance of dealing adequately with it. So, keeping his mind on the four risk-eliminating factors, he approaches the doctor with his hypothetical problem. He can even add another factor. He can tell the doctor that he is doing this for a class assignment, and that if the doctor resents the approach, the nurse is really not to blame. The instructor is at fault.

The most important reason for speaking to the doctor is that there is no substitute for actually taking the step and talking to a "superior." Trying the behavior must be an early step in the process of changing relationships. It is only after we have tried it that we can analyze what happened and begin to think of how we can make this behavior— or viable alternative behaviors—an integral part of our interaction with people. Let us look at some of the experiences that student nurses have had with this assignment.

One doctor said he hoped a nurse would feel free to let him know if he ever did anything wrong, as long as she didn't tell him in front of the patient. He added: "You're so busy sometimes, you don't know that you're doing something you shouldn't. Somebody has to tell you." The student was forced to revise her view that the only way to deal with a doctor was through her own supervisor. Just incidentally, the doctor offered the observation that if he saw a nurse doing something wrong, he would tell her, too. "You would talk to her directly and not to the head nurse?" the student asked him. "Right," he answered. "She might not know she is doing something wrong, and telling the head nurse might get her into trouble. And if I don't tell her, she'll never learn."

One student asked three different doctors about the hypothetical situation. One doctor said that the nurse should walk right up to the doctor and "ask him directly why he was avoiding the patient—regardless of a subsequent bad relationship between them." He explained that the welfare of the patient came first and interpersonnel relationships were of secondary importance.

The second doctor said that it was none of the nurse's business and that he would not want anyone interfering with him and his patients. He felt that any doctor must have a good reason for doing what he was doing. And, anyhow, no one should interfere with the work of a superior.

The third doctor said that whatever the nurse did would have to depend on the specific situation: the general competence of the doctor, the doctor's conscious decision to keep the patient unaware of his imminent death, the emotional state of the family, and so on.

The student was forced to conclude that she must avoid deciding what to do on the basis of any preconception of how doctors in general respond. She saw that each individual was just that—an individual—and every individual relationship is unique.

A physician from India revealed in an interview that his answer now would be quite different from what he would have said when he first came from India one year ago. He had come with the belief that women were in a subservient position to men, and that it would be presumptuous for any woman to tell a man that he was doing something wrong. (The student nurse was a woman and did not think to ask what his opinion would be if the nurse were a man, or the doctor a woman.) In his first months in the United States, he had assumed that the easy familiarity of Americans was a sign of disrespect and he maintained a rigid aloofness, especially in the hospital. He has since changed his view, and has even come so far as to feel that he would want a nurse to call his attention to a patient's needs—if she did so "respectfully."

Of course, if there were a functioning health team, this kind of one-to-one rapprochement would rarely be necessary. When a level of trust is built up in the course of the health team's functioning, concerns relating to the behavior and attitudes of its constituent personnel can be brought out at the regular meetings. Over a period of time, it becomes easier for a nurse to ask the reasons for a doctor's behavior without feeling that she is putting her head on the block.

This kind of experience, however, may be good *preparation* for becoming a member of a health team. If a nurse has many and varied experiences speaking as an equal, not only to doctors, but to head nurses, supervisors, and administrators, she need not fall into the trap of deferring to other medical personnel on the team because she feels she she must "keep her place." Thus, the health team never becomes a place where one hears lectures and gets patient assignments—that is, if there is a health team functioning at all.

If there is no health team in the hospital in which the nurse finds herself, she can get experience with peer-level interaction with all medical personnel, develop confidence in her professional ability and judgment, and come to believe that all medical personnel have equally important contributions to make to patient care. All this will give her the skills and initiative she needs so that she may finally take the leadership in establishing functioning health teams.

SUGGESTED INTERDISCIPLINARY EXPERIENCES

1. Identify the member of another health service whom you like, or admire, or would like to know better, or just feel comfortable with, so that the initial interdisciplinary experience may be somewhat easier to enter upon. Suggest to that person that for one week you spend a least two hours of the working day together. Try to spend most of those two hours working with patients for whom you both have some responsibility. This activity will probably be much easier for student nurses, since schedules and assignments can be arranged more easily to provide for optimum learning experiences. However, the graduate nurse can usually identify a physician, a dietitian, or an aide with whom to work for several hours in close collaboration, since every patient has some contact with other members of the health professions during his hospital stay.

Put it to the other person that you are interested in working out strategies for maximizing the effects of interdisciplinary cooperation in patient care. You might also suggest that the first step is to learn more about the other profession, so that you do not inadvertently interfere with the other's functioning or neutralize your own efforts.

Before you work with a patient, make some notes about what you see as the patient's needs and how you can administer to those needs. (Perhaps your colleague would like to do the same thing from his point of view. However, the most you can do is to tell him what you are doing; you cannot tell him what he should do!)

After you have worked together with the patient, spend a few

minutes discussing the patient, what has been done, how you think the
patient responded, what you see as additional patient needs that you
both may be able to provide for.

Continue to work together with this patient and to have your brief
discussions afterwards. At the end of the week, write a report of how
you perceive the patient's needs, what you have done to satisfy them,
and what you still feel you must do. Now take out your original diagnosis
and compare the two, answering these questions: (1) What needs did
you miss the first time? (2) Did working with the other professional help
you to make your own functioning more effective? Identify the specific
things you did that you might not have done if you were working alone
and say how they affected the patient. Identify the things you did not do
that you probably would have done if you were working alone. (3) Did
working with the other professional make your own functioning less
effective? (4) What were your feelings at working so closely with another
professional?

Another week, pick a member of another profession and repeat the
process. Perhaps after this experience, the other two people would like
to repeat the process, but with a larger team. This time, three of you
can work together, comparing your effectiveness before and after the experience. It is possible that you may find it so profitable and exhilarating,
that you will want to continue to add members of the various health
professions until you have an active interdisciplinary team working in
your department.

2. At lunch one day (if you eat in a hospital dining room or
cafeteria), instead of taking your tray to the table where all the student
nurses or the nurses sit, take it to the table where the aides or the medical
technicians or the interns sit. Since this takes some courage (breaking
social taboos are often more difficult than charting new courses in professional functioning), perhaps you can work in pairs. The people at the
table will rarely make any overt objection to your intrusion. (Let us not
mince words—you will probably be seen as intruders, and you will
probably also feel that you are; but we have been taught to be polite,
so you probably will not be told to leave.) So sit down, have your lunch,
smile and nod at the things that are said but say very little yourselves.
Do not talk to each other; this will tend to isolate you even more from
the other people.

Afterward, when you see the other people who were sitting at the
table, you will be able to smile in recognition, and even stop to talk
about something. Perhaps the next time you are in the cafeteria, it will be
more natural for you to sit together.

What is the point of all this? Like any other form of segregation,
the social separation of the health professions fosters intergroup misconceptions, at the very least, and hostility and fear at the other extreme. There

really does not seem to be any way of eliminating the misconceptions and developing positive, accepting feelings without making contact and beginning to communicate across group lines. But people must take the initial steps for making such contact; there is no alternative, no short-cut to communication. Those among us who are convinced of the necessity for working together, or are at least curious about exploring the possibilities for doing so, must somehow muster the courage to do something other than merely hoping for change. Sometimes we discover that the risk does not pay off—we encounter resistance and rejection. But those who are willing to take another risk, will find that—beyond the wall—there are others like themselves who also want to make contact, and they are welcomed.

Of course, the student nurse always has, as the ace up her sleeve, the justification that lets her off the hook—and considerably reduces her feeling of risk. She can always say that she is doing another one of those nutty assignments that characterize any formal educational experience. And she is doing it because her grade depends on it!

3. Here is something that should not be very difficult to do, because it really fits right in with the sort of thing we have done all through our school lives. Suppose that your class in nurse-patient relationships has spent two or three weeks working on a series of small-group projects. One group has explored the problems of caring for paraplegic patients. Another has gathered information and developed strategies for helping patients who know they are dying. Still another has studied the needs of children in hospitals. You are planning to meet as a class and share what you have learned. Each group has developed a different kind of presentation, ranging all the way from poems about dying to role-playing the sexual advances of a man who is paralyzed from the waist down.

Ask your instructor to invite to the presentations hospital personnel from the various professions. Invite some yourselves. Tell them all to feel free about raising questions and making comments after each presentation. Also make it clear that the name of the game is positive acceptance. Criticism—if it is absolutely necessary—is offered *lovingly*. And, unless there is in a presentation some gross error of fact, adverse criticism is deemed unnecessary. This takes away some of the natural anxiety of getting up in front of a group. Anyhow, most adverse criticism seems more to fulfill a personality need of the critic, rather than to assist in the learning process of the people criticized. It is really totally irrelevant that the acting in role-playing is not of movie star quality, or that a description of a child's behavior is not the way *most* children respond. For purposes of the presentation, the role-playing is merely an opportunity to substitute simulation for words, which does not require professional actors. And the fact that *most* children do not respond in a certain way, does not reduce the importance of the fact that *some* children do, and that medical personnel must be prepared to deal with those children too.

Perhaps, after the presentations and discussion, you may suggest that you would appreciate invitations to lectures in other departments when the subject matter seems pertinent to the improvement of nursing care. When such interchange becomes an accepted part of the hospital's educational program, the atmosphere exists for approaching patient care from an interdisciplinary point of view.

Now that you have had a number of experiences with people in the other health professions, here is an opportunity to clarify your point of view.

Below are five points of view about a nurse's relationship with the members of the other health services. Pick the point of view that is closest to what you believe and change the wording until it says exactly what you think. Or you may write a new point of view that is your own. The idea is to be able to get a paragraph about which you can say, "This is my belief."

When you have decided where you stand, you may share your opinions with one another, plan additional experiences for yourself, or simply put the whole matter into the back of your mind for a while, to think about again in a month or two.

> 1. The job of the nurse is to follow out the orders of the doctor and the nursing supervisor. It is not within the nurse's province to question the professional judgments of the people in charge.
>
> 2. The nurse, as a health practitioner, is not only competent to make professional judgments, but he has a *responsibility* to do so. If he sees something wrong being done to a patient, he must intercede and prevent any possible injury to the patient. Of course, like every professional, when he makes a judgment he assumes responsibility for any error he makes.
>
> 3. The nurse's job is nursing care. What the doctor and other personnel do is not her responsibility. However, if she knows that another nurse is not doing her job properly, she has a responsibility to do something about it.
>
> 4. Too much frankness among the various health workers—doctors, nurses, aides—causes constant turmoil. Everyone should mind his own business and do his own job and be courteous to others. This will maintain in the hospital that atmosphere of calm professionalism that patients need if they are to have confidence in the people caring for them.
>
> 5. It is not the professional thing to do to criticize your colleagues. Of course, if a sub-professional is doing something wrong—or just not doing the job—then the nurse must do something about it.

9 *THE STUDENT NURSE*

REASONS FOR CHOOSING NURSING

The student nurse comes to her chosen profession for various reasons. Always there has been the romance of the profession that has lured young women. The cool, white-clad vision with the warm heart is a lovely picture in many minds and is often the focus of the dreams of young girls. Today, TV shows foster this picture, and not inconsequentially add to it the very cogent possibility of marrying a handsome young physician.

There is, at the same time, the prestige of being a nurse, with all the respect given to a member of the health professions in our society. Students are often surprised at how, in social situations, friends approach them with all kinds of health questions, hanging on their answers as if they were consulting highly qualified specialists. They even ask questions that their own physicians have already answered for them, and it is not unusual for them to give more credence to the response of the student—someone in whom they vest all the trust that goes with personal friendship.

Some young people go into nursing largely because it is a means of leaving home. This is no small matter in an era when leaving home is an essential part of the youth culture, even though the risks and difficulties attendant upon leaving the comfort and security of home are many. Going into nursing—like going away to college—becomes an opportunity to exchange the security of home for the security of a "program" in which meals are prepared, a bed is provided, and there is the comfort to be had from living with a number of peers who are sharing the same situational problems.

The most important reason for entering nursing for most people is the desire to give service in the particular ways that nursing does. The opportunity to alleviate pain, speed healing, and give comfort during the whole illness and recuperation process is one that appeals very much to most student nurses. And today, with the growing emphasis on the role of the nurse in education and the prevention of illness, the prospect of service becomes even more attractive for many.

SPECIAL NEEDS

Student nurses face many fears as they enter upon their new career. In the rush to fulfill all the requirements of the program, these fears usually receive no official recognition. They have a tendency to become the topic of grousing and other forms of conversation among the students, but little is done to work them through and deal with them productively.

First, there are the fears associated with the academic requirements. There are some who have the idea that these are rather easy, especially in three-year programs. More and more students are finding that the academic standards in nursing programs are not very different from those in the undergraduate programs of other disciplines. Not only are the physical sciences dealt with rigorously, but psychology and sociology are studied in some depth. And the usual demands that students modify their interpersonal relations are changing from exhortations to be "professional" and informal pressures to "adjust" into a rubric of formal opportunities for self-analysis and change.

The resulting tensions often seem to have effects on the physical health of students. I always get the feeling that there are more colds, flus, digestive upsets, and even more serious illnesses among student nurses than among other students. And every illness—no matter how minor—raises the level of fear that ground will be lost in studying, examinations will be missed, and it will be impossible to make it all up.

Socially, student nurses are beset with the same feelings that other students experience. Away from home for the first time, thrown in with strangers, all of whom, at first sight, seem more self-assured, more popular, more capable of coping than she is, the student begins to feel that her reasons for becoming a nurse were, perhaps, not so valid. As with most students in most schools, there seems to be a sink-or-swim philosophy, and—except for an occasional movie or lecture or dance—the students grasp at their own opportunities for a social life.

How poignant are these comments by students who have been in a university nursing program for about two months:

"I have learned to eat food that is not like mother's," says one with all the yearning of a child who feels far from home.

And another says stoically, "As far as living with other girls is concerned, I haven't learned much except to wait for the bathtub, even if I have to wait for two hours."

To the usual social problems are added some that many students never encounter, since they attended schools that still operate as if the world were not changing. In many of the schools of nursing, Black applicants are being assiduously recruited, and it is not unusual for a Black and a white nurse to find themselves as roommates. Certainly Black and white students are often assigned to the same service and must work together. And both Black and white students must care for patients of of the other race.

Since most of us—both Black and white—live within our own groups, with minimal equal-status contact with members of other groups, students need to learn, in the face of all the errors they have learned about other races, how to live and work together amicably. This is no small adjustment to make in a society like ours.

To all of these pressures are added the interpersonal/professional stresses that arise in the student's contact with the teachers of nursing and the director of nursing services. The nursing service head, who is concerned primarily with providing adequate nursing care for patients, often comes into conflict with the nursing instructor, who is concerned that the student get the kind of clinical experience that will help him become a competent nurse. Sometimes these two objectives are in apparent conflict, and the resultant sparks that fly are likely to burn the student— a relatively innocent bystander.

Certainly both the nursing service and the nursing education people do equally important jobs. Why, then, the conflict? There seems to be, in both people, a fear that their job will not get done. There never seems to be an adequate enough staff to give all the necessary patient care. Similarly, there never seems to be enough time to teach a student everything he must know. The people responsible for doing these jobs inevitably feel tense and frustrated, and may very well take it out on one another— to say nothing of taking it out on the student!

Nor are the tension and frustration they feel unrelated to some very practical considerations. If they fail on the job, their financial and professional security can go down the drain, as do all the satisfactions that go with successful accomplishment.

There are also those who fight for prestige, power, and domination, always at the expense of those around them. Fighting for the right to control the student—his time, his assignments, his loyalty—is often a part of the conflict. The result can be a fearful student, with increasing difficulty in learning. The students' fear and frustration can not only affect their ability to learn, but they may—unable to vent their hostility on the people who are causing it—become resigned and apathetic, doing only the minimum amount of work needed to get by. Or they may displace their hostility onto others—peers and patients—in ways that are not always easy to detect and prevent.

Student nurses have some problems relating to graduate nurses in general. Sometimes, when the graduate nurse and the student are working side by side, it is easy for the graduate to forget that the other person *is* only a student, with limited training and experience. Expectations of what she can do are often too great. Each time the student falls short of what is unrealistically expected of her, she is made to feel a failure. Even if nothing is said to her, her own evaluation of herself is made in terms of what others expect of her.

Finally, we cannot overlook the feelings that are generated in student nurses when it begins to come clear to them that most of their expectations of nursing as a profession are only illusions. The romance rarely exists, the prestige is overshadowed by feelings of inadequacy and powerlessness, and the service often goes unappreciated.

UNIQUE CONTRIBUTIONS

But in spite of these difficulties, people come to nursing with some strengths that should be recognized and carefully preserved by the profession that trains them. The most important strength is one that instructors and supervisors immediately set about neutralizing: Student nurses have a great desire to become involved with people. They *care* about those who suffer, and they want to nurture and help. However, almost from the first day of their training period they are admonished that becoming emotionally involved is unprofessional, and so their enthusiasm for essential human touching is slowly but surely diminished as they fall into line with the demands of the school and the hospital.

Student nurses are gregarious. They enjoy other people and like to be with them. Here again, the profession is taking people with a special and valuable trait and training it out of them. The shift of emphasis in nursing practice from patient care to everything *except* patient care makes some of us contemplate the waste with dismay.

Many young people these days are eager to let their involvement carry them into roles of leadership. They are frequently willing to become change agents, with all the risks involved. Nursing education, perhaps more than other areas of post-high school education, very often evaluates students and defines their success in terms of conformity and unquestioning compliance. In spite of this, the National Student Nurses Association has active chapters in forty-three states. It has made special efforts to reach high school students who need special help if they are to fulfill their ambition to become nurses—students who are poor, those who have attended inferior schools and so need tutoring, those who have experienced discrimination because of race or nationality.

I think student nurses and young people generally need more freedom to become everything that their teachers have never been able to be. In spite of the hysterical diatribes against permissiveness and the conviction of many adults that young people need more restraints placed upon them, I see much youthful behavior in quite a different light. If young people smoke marijuana and take pills to change their moods, they are merely emulating the significant adults in their lives who demonstrate the same behavior even though they use different drugs. Young people have never learned to free themselves of these adult responses to the stresses of living. If young people grab for simplistic solutions to the complex problems of contemporary life—solutions like fundamentalism or artsy-craftsy communalism—they are merely repeating my generation's reliance on the two or three easily identified supports for security. We called it a house, a car, and a bank account, and we felt satisfied and safe. They call it Jesus, Hari Krishna or working with your hands, and they feel satisfied, safe, *and* superior to their parents. There is no generation gap for many young people: the generations are mirror images of each other.

Fortunately, there are many young people who really are breaking away from old, destructive, uncreative modes of life. Those of us who have the courage will help them do it.

THE CLASSROOM AS A SAFETY VALVE AND AN ARENA FOR PLANNING CHANGE

Beset by pressures both internal and external, the student nurse needs some mechanism for dealing with such pressures in systematically productive ways. A classroom really devoted to the education of the whole student can provide such a mechanism. There, in relative safety, he can express his feelings, sort out the parameters of his problems, and try out ways of solving them. Much of the frustration that comes from random and circular griping and a feeling that one has no power to change things can be alleviated by involvement in planning for change.

There is, of course, some threat to faculty and hospital staff in encouraging students to consider alternatives in the education of themselves. However, as a faculty member, I have always considered it far safer to take an active part in the change process rather than be the casualty in a violent revolution I have tried to hold back. (There are no other choices: there will be change, one way or another.)

There have been times when I have come to a class prepared with lectures and activities for a two- or three-hour session. After the first five minutes, I have become aware of an unusual restlessness or an undercurrent of tension that indicated something disturbing was happening to people. I could, of course, go on with my prepared agenda and afterward feel comfortable about having "covered" the necessary material. But I have learned that the teacher's "teaching" is not the objective. The goal is the student's learning. So I have abandoned the plans and set the scene for dealing with the immediate problem:

1. I have said to a class of forty students, "You are upset about something. Do you want to talk about it?"

2. Those students who are able to speak freely burst out in a rush of feeling:

> "The chemistry instructor is unfair."
>
> "He doesn't know what he's doing!"
>
> "He can't teach, so he takes it out on us!"
>
> "Who needs all that stuff anyhow? It doesn't help us to be good nurses. It's just for taking tests!"

Other students nod agreement. Some, by the looks on their faces, do not agree, but they say nothing.

3. After five minutes of this, I observe aloud that perhaps it would help everyone get a chance to speak if the class broke up into small groups. I suggest that each group might want to spell out the problem— or problems— in writing. If, in the process of defining the problem, questions are raised to which they do not have the answers, they ought to write down those questions, too. They have about thirty minutes for this. (This is usually time enough to express their feelings, since they have probably been expressing strong feelings to one another in informal settings outside of class. The time is limited enough so that they must soon pull themselves from the wholesale condemnations and begin to focus on the job of defining the problem.)

4. As each group completes its talk, one person in the group writes on a sheet of chart paper the problem—or problems—as that group sees them. He also writes the questions to which they do not have answers. The charts are put up on the wall where everyone can see them.

5. The first thing the class notices is that not all the groups have

listed the same problems or the same questions. For example, Group 1 says that the instructor doesn't know how to cover the required material in the allotted time, so he resorts to simply telling students to learn the material in the book and gives them frequent tests. Group 2 says the required material has no relation to effective nursing, and they should not have to learn it. Group 3 raises the question, "Is the required material needed by nurses?" Group 4 has jumped the gun. They want the instructor fired for incompetence.

6. Someone suggests that they need the answers to the questions before they can agree on what the problems are. Small committees and individuals select the questions they find most interesting. They ask for class time to plan strategy for getting the answers. While the rest of the class is role-playing communication with patients (now they appear ready for this step, since they have taken steps to solve the immediate problem) the ten volunteers work in a group apart. They ask me how one goes about checking on the relevance of chemistry facts to effective nursing practice. I suggest that they take two or three of the facts at random and try to see if they are needed in any of the clinical experiences they have had in the past two weeks. Two of them take this suggestion. Another student decides to compare last week's lecture notes in chemistry with the last three chapters in the nursing practices textbook. Two students say they will interview nurses on the floor and get their point of view. Another will—hesitantly—approach the chemistry instructor to find out if *he* sees any connection between chemistry and nursing.

Everyone promises to bring the results of the research to the next class session.

7. Next time, the researchers reveal their discovery that knowledge of some chemistry facts are obviously essential to specific nursing tasks. They conjecture that other facts may be equally important in ways they do not know as yet. They wonder if they may re-define the problem with their instructor: How to learn chemistry so that the connection with nursing is apparent as the course progresses. The student who interviewed the instructor volunteers the information that he knows very little about nursing, but that he is apaprently a competent chemist. He has a Ph.D. in the subject and has written many articles for professional journals. When she asked him how he decided what to include in a chemistry course for nurses, he answered that the course he gave was the usual undergraduate introductory course in chemistry. This is what the nursing department had asked him to teach.

She added, for the edification of her fellow students, "He's really not a bad guy once you get to talk to him. He comes through real human."

8. The class rallies almost spontaneously around a new definition of the problem: How can chemistry be made a real part of *nursing*

education? I suggest that this is a good time to use brainstorming. Each person takes a stack of small papers and writes his ideas—one to a paper—on how to solve this problem. All the papers are collected.

9. In small groups again, they sort out the ideas, discarding some, combining others, and deciding on two or three as most feasible.

10. A committee made up of two representatives from each group takes the final eight or ten ideas and develops them into a plan for solving the problem.

11. The plan is presented to the whole class and, with minor modifications, is put into operation.

The Plan

1. Since the chemistry instructor admits that he does not know much about nursing, we will have to take the initiative in making chemistry relevant to our needs.

2. Get the instructor to agree to devote some class time to explaining the connection between chemistry and nursing. Since he is worried about covering the curriculum, we will promise in exchange to be responsible for learning the required material.

3. At the end of each class session, one of us or a group demonstrates a connection between chemical information learned the previous week and a nursing technique. For such demonstrations, we are free to enlist the aid of anyone in any of the health professions.

4. We reserve the right to insist that the instructor remain for these demonstrations, so that classes that come after ours don't have to go through what we've had to.

One look at the plan and it becomes clear that the students' agitation and near rebellion was *not* caused by their reluctance to work or any desire to avoid responsibility. Overworked and anxious as they often were about the new experiences they were having, the apparent meaninglessness of this one course was just the final straw. It became the target for all their frustrations. The sense of being at the mercy of an institution that seemed to care nothing about their feelings added to their sense of powerlessness and intensified their need to exercise some control over their own fate. They had to feel that the system was responsive to their needs.

This is not the only or necessarily the best way to use the classroom for solving a pressing problem of a group of students. It is possible that, once exposed to this procedure, the students will adapt it to suit their purposes much better. However, the method implicitly makes the suggestion that people have a right to—and can—take control of their own lives. And they can do so without destroying themselves or others.

The information-gathering and problem-solving sessions, as well as the ultimate implementation of the plan, seemed to have immediate effects on the students. They certainly were more interested in chemistry and, although this result was not systematically substantiated, I would venture an educated guess that they learned more chemistry and remembered it for a longer time than do students exposed to the traditional lecture/examination process. Certainly their active participation and the inclusion of health personnel in the course reduced the level of boredom for them.

But I think the longer-term results were even more significant. These students learned that they can successfully take a hand in their own education. They had experience in changing a situation they believed was unchangeable. They learned to use the resources available in the profession to do a job better, and they were surprised to discover that no one was ever so detached or uninterested that he would not respond to a request for help. Before the semester was over, more doctors, nurses, dieticians, and aides felt involved in the education of this class than had ever before cared about what was happening in the class. Professional associations formed between students and other staff have remained to this day.

DEALING WITH
INDIVIDUAL PROBLEMS

Students are caught up in their own problems of survival and often are not even aware that some of their number are in imminent danger of going down for the third time. The classroom in which the level of trust is high, in which students and teacher are not afraid to share their experiences, express their feelings and make errors, is a place where people are not afraid to ask for help. The teacher can, at the outset, institute mechanisms that make asking for help a normal part of group interaction.

Here is a technique that students may find useful. Have the class break up into triads. In each group of three people, one is *A,* one is *B* and one is *C.*

1. *A* tells about a problem he is facing and with which he can use some help.

2. *B* gives help.

3. *C* gives his opinion of how effective or useful *B*'s help is.

4. *B* tells about a problem *he* is facing, *C* gives help, and *A* gives feedback on the usefulness of the help.

5. *C* tells about a problem, *A* gives help, and *B* provides feedback.

If this exercise is done often enough, students get into the habit of asking for help. They also become more skillful in giving it.

Recently, I had a very satisfying experience in helping students that grew out of a need to cope with an unsatisfactory situation. I walked into a room to meet my new class, and I saw fifty-eight students sitting and looking at me, ready for "the word." I did a rapid mental shuffle and made a decision. I told them that I thought they could accomplish more if they were able to work in smaller groups. Consequently, I was asking them to break up into groups of not more than ten people. I strongly suggested that, since this was a course that dealt with intergroup relations, it would be useful for each small group to include members of various social groups—race, sex, and age particularly; regional and professional where possible.

They began grouping themselves immediately and quickly, apparently intrigued with this novel opening to a graduate course. They joked about such things as swapping a man for any white person, setting the tone of easy interaction that was never lost. Almost at once the groups began to call themselves "families," and individuals said again and again how comfortable it was to come to a "family" of ten each session and be welcomed and enfolded, rather than to come into a class of fifty-eight, unrecognized.

The students became so close to the other members of their "family" that they almost naturally helped one another in difficult situations. The danger of developing habits of "sibling rivalry" was discussed openly, but it was generally prevented because students became convinced that each one of them had something valuable to offer and that there was nothing to be gained from competing with one another.

Usually, faculty members know when a student is failing and offer extra help or lectures on shaping up. It might be worthwhile to ask the student if he would like the help of his classmates. Sometimes a caring instructor can ease the way for a reluctant student to avail himself of the assistance of his peers. The instructor may even—with the permission and involvement of the troubled student—arrange for an informal meeting with three or four receptive students to explore possibilities for such assistance.

Some of the small-group discussions might profitably revolve around such questions as, "Why do students flunk out of nursing programs?" and "What are some of the things classmates can do to prevent such failures?" "What are some of the reasons why a student might decide nursing is not for him?" and "How might he involve his classmates in helping him come to the best decision?"

Sometimes, even while all the efforts are being made to develop openness and trust, a device can be used for preserving the anonymity of people in difficulties. Anyone needing some possible answers to a question or some alternative solutions to a problem may want to put the request into a "Problem Box" or post it on a bulletin board. Then the class can be encouraged to take the initiative in exploring the problems (by role-playing or any other technique) or discussing the questions during regular class sessions. The anonymous student thus may profit from the thinking of the group and may even have the chance to practice some of the suggested behaviors without having publicly to identify the problem as his.

These techniques for caring and helping have very specific professional implications for the nurse. The problems confronting nurses that have been discussed in this book are complex and difficult to cope with. Forced to face them alone, many of us in defense encapsulate ourselves in armor of denial and indifference and go through life only half involved, half alive. To put out a helping hand is also to feel the responsive touch of another human being, and there is nothing else in the world more encouraging.

Nurses can help one another to ease the sorrow of pain and death. They can take turns reminding others of the successes of the profession and the strengths of its practitioners, so that nobody, in a period of discouragement, is abandoned to self-recriminations. They can support and sustain one another in their battles against ignorance and brutality. And they can enjoy one another because each one sees himself reflected in his colleague's success.

10 *COMMUNICATING WITH THE PATIENT*

PRACTICING COMMUNICATION

Find one other person to work with. Each member of the couple takes turns playing the patient and the nurse. In each one of the following situations, only the person playing the patient gets the script. The person playing the nurse tries to provide what she thinks the patient needs or wants.

After each situation is played, the "patient" tells the nurse how close she came to complying with the patient's wishes. Keep score of the number of successes you have as a couple. (The patient alone makes the final decision on what is success.)

Situation 1

You are a middle-aged woman in the hospital for the first time. You have lived alone for all of your adult life, and one of the most disturbing factors in the prospect of an extended stay in the hospital is the necessity of giving up your cherished privacy. You have managed to get a private room, and you want to keep the door closed at all times. The nurses, the aides, and even the doctors seem bent on (1) leaving the door

159

open each time they come and go, (2) "encouraging" you to leave it open so you can see people, (3) teasing you about being unfriendly, and so on, all because they believe that you would be better off if you did not keep your door closed. You are trying to make the charge nurse understand how you feel so she can help you maintain your privacy.

Situation 2

You are a man in your middle twenties and you are feeling very uncomfortable even though your illness is not serious. It bothers you very much to be flat on your back and out of commission; this conflicts with your image of yourself as a strong, self-sufficient individual who "never had a sick day in my life." You don't want your friends and relatives to see you this way, but you can't get anyone to put a *no visitors* sign on your door. You are trying to convince the nurse to tell people you are not having visitors.

Situation 3

You have just been told that you have a very serious illness. Although the doctor hasn't said so, you know enough to realize that you will die very soon. You need to be alone to come to grips with this thing. (You have always preferred to be alone when faced with a crisis.) Everyone seems bent on "keeping you company" and "cheering you up." You are trying to convince the nurse that you want to be left completely alone.

Situation 4

You are very much afraid that the surgery you are scheduled to undergo within the next two days will leave you severely handicapped. No matter how many times the doctor and the nurses tell you that you are unnecessarily concerned, you are not convinced. You need repeated reassurance that you will be all right, but you are not the sort of person to ask outright for such assurance, or to put your consuming fear into words. The best you can do is to keep saying—in different ways—that you will never fully recover. Each time you say this, what you hope is that the nurse will tell you again that you will be all right. You are going through the process of saying you will be crippled and hoping for reassurance for the twentieth time today.

Situation 5

You are a woman of about forty who has just undergone serious surgery. You are now awake and only mildly uncomfortable, although you must lie flat on your back and cannot move easily. The doctor has ordered complete quiet and no visitors, but nobody seems to understand that the quiet and isolation is terrifying to you. You have a large family— brothers, sisters, cousins—as well as five children of your own. In times of trouble, everybody rallies round to offer advice, solace, and just company. Everybody talks at once, and, to an outsider, it seems like bedlam. But to the family it is the very stuff of life. Now, alone and in silence, you feel overwhelmed with a growing feeling of doom that you cannot shake. You are trying to convince the nurse that you must have your family around you or you will surely die.

COMMUNICATION SKILLS

Usually, when we study communication skills, we are concerned with developing the ability to communicate our thoughts and feelings to others. Too often, we are so intent on our own need to communicate that we overlook the fact that communication is a shared process. The professional—the teacher, the nurse—recognizes that part of the skill in communication involves the ability to help others communicate with us. For without information from our students and our patients, we cannot function effectively. We are taught that we must deal with each patient in terms of his unique needs; however, we cannot acquire this talent simply by reading the chapter on individual needs in the textbook. We must find ways of helping each patient communicate his needs to us. In each one of these cases, there is no doubt that the patient must assume part of the responsibility for getting his needs attended to. He must make himself understood; he must communicate his needs to others. However, it behooves the professional to be aware of the difficulties of human com- munication and the many psychological obstacles that prevent us from stating openly and clearly what we want. After awareness, the nurse needs (1) skills in aiding the patient to communicate his needs, and (2) skills in interpreting what the patient is trying to communicate without words.

AIDING THE PATIENT TO COMMUNICATE HIS NEEDS

Direct Questioning

How are we to help another person let us know what he wants us to know about him? Of course, we can always question

him directly: What would you like me to do for you? How can I
help you? Would you like to tell me what is on your mind? These are all
open questions that indicate that the nurse is aware that the patient wants
something, but that she has no idea what it is that he does want. If the
patient is afraid or embarrassed to say what he wants, or if he does not
know exactly what he wants but knows only that he has certain feelings,
such questions may not be helpful to him. Such questions *are* helpful if the
patient merely needs an unstructured opportunity and a ready ear to
express his needs.

Recognition of Feelings

For the person who is filled with feelings and cannot
focus them enough to ask for help, the nurse may encourage him to
express those feelings as a first step in identifying the needs. She
may say, "You seem to have some strong feelings of frustration."
*And then she must be quiet and listen attentively to any response the
patient may make.* Often, all that a person needs is some encouragement
to express his feelings. After the feelings are all out in the open, he may
get to what he wants of the people around him. The important thing is for
the nurse to listen without judging or evaluating, without giving advice
or scolding. For example, there is little calculated to increase the level
of frustration more than to be told—oh so soothingly—"You shouldn't feel
that way." The point is, the way a person feels is an unarguable fact and
must be accepted without question or judgment. Steps may be taken to
help the person feel differently but *telling* him to do so is not, to say the
least, very helpful.

Offering Multiple Choices

When a nurse has some clues about what the patient wants,
she may give him further help. She may offer him a number
of choices from which he may find it easy to identify what he has
not been able to communicate. For example, the nurse may have identified,
in the outpouring of feelings, a general area of concern: relationships
with medical personnel. However, she is not sure exactly what the problem
is. Rather than taking a chance and making a wrong diagnosis (and
thereby perhaps causing the patient to withdraw completely), she may
say: "Patients often have problems in relating to nurses and doctors. Sometimes, doctors and nurses don't seem to have time to listen to patients and
find out what is bothering them. Sometimes medical people seem almost

rude when they talk to each other about the patient, and say little or nothing to the patient. Patients are sometimes afraid to insist on getting attention, because they don't want to be thought overdemanding."

Given a number of choices, a patient may feel somewhat freer to identify *his* choice when he realizes that other people face similar problems and that nurses are aware of the problems and are not given to negative judgments of individuals who have these problems.

Enlisting Other Assistance

Sometimes, nothing the nurse or doctor can do is helpful in facilitating the patient's communication, although he is obviously laboring under the burden of urgent and unmet needs. One must consider that the patient's perception of the doctor and nurse is what is interfering with his ability to communicate. The perceived chasm between him and the professional may be too great for him to breach, and no amount of reassurance or skill can close that breach. The nurse would be wise, here, to enlist the aid of another person to help the patient verbalize his needs. Here an aide or an orderly may be able to make the patient more comfortable in conversation; a member of his own family may be easier to communicate with; even a member of his own race, or religion, or sex may encourage him to confide his problems. However, no matter whom the nurse asks for help, nothing must be done without the patient's full knowledge. That is, it must be made clear to the patient that what he confides to an aide will be communicated to people who can meet his needs, unless he specifically denies permission to do this. If permission is denied in advance, then the prospective confidante must make up her own mind about whether or not she wants to accept the communication. She may decide that she will listen to the patient only if she can tell the nurse what is troubling him. Whatever she decides, the patient must have the final choice of telling or not telling his problems.

The point is that the patient must not be deceived, misled, or manipulated by the people around him. If the basis of optimum communication is always mutual trust, then we must foster this trust. Deception and manipulation are a denial of trust.

Providing Safety in Numbers

There is nothing like getting group support to give one a feeling of safety. To provide such safety, the nurse may encourage a number of patients to discuss their unmet needs and decide how best to inform the hospital staff of these needs. All the patients in the same room may make up the group, or perhaps the "group" may be only the two patients in adjacent beds. Ambulatory patients from several rooms may be brought in to make up a group.

The nurse may say to several patients, "Sometimes people feel very helpless in a hospital. They need things but they don't know how to go about getting what they need. You may find it easier to discuss your needs with one another and then let me know as a group what I can do for you."

Clues in Interpreting Non-verbal Communication

When words will not come, or if they are used to mask real feelings, then there are clues to the meanings of non-verbal communication that may help the nurse "read" the patient accurately. The person who automatically answers, "Fine" to a question about how he feels needs additional encouragement to speak about his condition. His response may very well be a "polite" one, designed not to give information, but to return a greeting. It may be prompted by what you are communicating to him. If your question is always brisk and brief and your manner makes it clear that you have stopped only for a moment midway between two very important activities, he may feel that you do not really want the answer to your question.

The patient who talks about everything except his illness, himself, and his immediate family may be too frightened to put his situation into words. He may need you to mention it first, wording your comment in such a way that he will be encouraged to continue the conversation: "This is your first time in a hospital, Mr. Smith, isn't it?"

The one who fits the stereotype of the ideal patient too perfectly also needs special help in communicating. Usually, what nurses do is congratulate themselves and one another on the patient who doesn't complain, doesn't keep asking for things, maintains self control, and generally gives them no trouble. This is not unlike the teacher whose quiet little student is slowly expiring under his unsolved problems. As long as medical personnel are not happy with "temperamental" patients, patients who cry when they are sad, scream when they hurt, and ask for company when they are lonely, there will be "model" patients. And as long as there are model patients, medical people will be able to fool themselves into thinking they are treating the whole person.

The patient who has given up trying to communicate because he speaks another language must not be permitted to remain silent. Surely in a cosmopolitan society such as ours, someone can be found who knows the language or is willing to learn a few sentences. Sometimes the

patient himself can be enlisted as the teacher and thus be provided with
a chance to reduce the discouragement and sense of helplessness caused
by being unable to communicate with those around him.

We know enough about some groups to realize that an individual
may be silent because he is very frightened, and we need to take steps to
encourage speaking. Children are often afraid that the child who is taken
from the ward and not returned must be dead, although they may never
mention it. Children also are afraid of what will happen to them while they
are asleep and helpless on the operating table. If you cannot get the child
to speak, you know enough about role-playing by now to help him act out
his feelings. For example, you can "play a game" with him, in which he is the
daddy and he is visting his son in the hospital. While you play the child,
listen carefully to the things "daddy" says: "They're not going to cut off
your tummy" (meaning "I am afraid that is what they are going to do to
me."), and "You will wake up and be fine" (meaning "I am afraid I am
going to die.").

THE PATIENT AS A PERSON

What we as a society seem to be trying to do is to divest ourselves
of our humanity. We number, catalogue, and computerize ourselves so
that we can maintain interpersonal communication at a minimum level.
Store clerks no longer interact with us to discover who we are, what we
like, and whether or not we can pay for the merchandise being sold. All
supermarkets have the meats displayed in the same part of the store,
and the produce is there for the picking and squeezing. Our credit ratings
quickly are established by punching a few buttons. (This only in certain
neighborhoods, of course. In other neighborhoods no personal checks are
accepted even though they could be as easily checked for validity. The
only checks accepted and even eagerly sought are welfare checks. Prices
are even raised on the days they are expected.)

Our social security cards display our numbers more prominently
than our names. Many places with which we do business answer no
inquiries about our accounts unless we identify ourselves by number.

In the name of technology and efficiency the patient, too, is often
dehumanized, reduced to a collection of parts that need maintenance and
repair. People who run large institutions like metropolitan hospitals need
constantly to weigh in the balance the benefits of efficiency and the needs
of humanity. There is such a thing as being too efficient, saving a dollar
by increasing a fear, or saving an hour and perpetuating loneliness.

The patient does not leave himself at the entrance to the hospital
while he abandons a set of symptoms to the ministrations of medical people

and the limitations of hospital routine. He brings with him his quite normal intelligence and his knowledge of medicine (which may not be inconsiderable, given the reams of writing and the hours of television viewing devoted to symptoms and treatments). He brings also his feelings, most of which are *not* immediately related to his illness, and his whole apperceptive mass that has been developed in terms of his group culture, his education, and all his life experiences up until the time of his admission into the hospital. Although his illness may be his most immediate and greatest concern, just how he expresses that concern in his feelings and behavior is a function of everything he is as a human being.

How, then, does one justify asking, "How do we feel today?" thus carelessly denying his individuality? How, also, does one explain the reference to him as "the appendectomy in Room 30" or "the CVA who was brought in last night," references that cancel him out as anything but the end result of his pathology?

Nor is this just being picky about semantics! The use of these words is merely symptomatic of the speaker's focus. She is not a bit concerned that she doesn't know Mr. Brown, as long as she is able to identify and treat the disease. Of course, medical people know—intellectually, at any rate—that a disease may be treated "efficiently" in such a way as to increase the patient's suffering and even cause his death.

I must say a word here about the almost universal practice of discussing a patient in his presence as if he were not really there. If anything is calculated to make an individual in *any* situation feel powerless and of little worth, it is hearing other people making observations about him and decisions to do things to him without ever acknowledging his presence. Medical people protest that the patient cannot understand the technical language anyway, or that orders need to be given quickly, but there seems to be more to it than that. Sometimes it seems as if doctors and nurses are merely trying to demonstrate their superiority over the patients. Sometimes it is clear that they think the patient is childlike and not capable of participating in adult conversation.

I was once told of a physician who gave an entering college student a routine examination and then *called her mother into the office to tell her the results of the examination.* Not once did he turn to the eighteen-year-old daughter to indicate that he thought she might be interested in what he had to say.

If physicians are more guilty of this kind of behavior than nurses are, then perhaps nurses need to resist abetting them. You know how to make a conversation between you and the doctor into a three-way discussion —even if all you do is turn occasionally to the patient and make eye contact. (It is well to remember that children, too, may dislike the feeling of being talked around and ignored.)

THE PATIENT'S FEELINGS

I tuned in recently to one of those hospital TV shows that abound these days and heard a bit of dialogue that seemed to exemplify a recurrent aspect of the pattern of interaction between patients and medical personnel. "I'm a little scared," the patient confided to the doctor. "Don't be scared," the doctor responded, and went on with the prescribed medical procedure. I had a similar personal experience not very long ago. Faced with the prospect of surgery, I hesitantly confided in the resident my fear of general anaesthesia. "I'm rather phobic about losing consciousness," I said, "and I'm so afraid that the anaesthetic will make me feel as if I'm fainting." "Everybody feels that way," he said brusquely, and left my room, leaving me to struggle alone with the fear that he had effectively intensified by the bit of information he had so casually proffered.

These two situations demonstrate, I think, much more than insensitivity to the patient's feelings. There actually seems to be an element of denial in the physicians' responses: It is as if they were saying, "Your feelings do not exist." It is difficult to understand the reasons for such an attitude. Can it be that the physician feels so much more competent in medical matters than he does when faced with psychological problems? Can he be avoiding dealing with feelings because his *own* feelings—of fear and of helplessness—stand in the way? Is there, perhaps, some cultural factor intervening: Does the male doctor, particularly, feel that it is somehow un-masculine for him to respond to a patient's feelings?

I have heard some male doctors laud the virtues of an LPN who was so "loving," so "feeling," so "nurturing." They always hastened to add that she had none of the technical or professional expertise of registered nurses, but they agreed that they preferred her to give nursing care rather than the best trained nurses. The implication always seemed to be that feelings and professional skill were somehow incompatible. Perhaps this is the belief that rationalizes a physician's avoidance of feelings.

There was a line in an old novel that also seemed to put this idea into words. A nurse was very moved at the suffering of a child in the hospital, and she cried. The physician rebuked her for being sentimental. When she accused him of being hard and unfeeling, he snarled at her: "I don't have to cry; I can *do* something to help the child. Crying is for those who can't do anything else!" He dismissed the suggestion that crying might be something other than merely an expression of helpless frustration —that it might be a way of communicating, of sharing feelings, of reaching out to another human being for mutual comfort and support.

Responding to the feelings of others means somehow communicating that you share those feelings. You cannot say to someone who is mourning, "I know how you feel," and use a flat, colorless, emotionless tone of voice. There must be some *matching* of emotional tone, or the patient will have no evidence that the nurse really does know how he feels.

ARE PATIENTS FREE?

We may be surprised to discover that many patients are afraid of hospital personnel. I do not mean that they are frightened about being sick, or about the treatments they must undergo. This, too, is frightening, of course, and understandably so. What I am talking about here is the kind of fear people have of other people that is the essence of captivity and enslavement. Patients are often afraid that, if they complain about what is happening to them in the hospital, they will be badly treated (in vague, unexplainable ways) in retaliation for their complaints. Some feel that if they make too many requests of hospital personnel, no one will answer their call when they are in serious difficulty and need help immediately.

To say that these fears are unfounded is really beside the point. They are the kinds of fears that are generated by feelings of powerlessness— whether the person is in a hospital or in any ordinary political-social situation. The point is that he finds himself in a repressive society, at the mercy of the people in power. He feels that he must play a completely submissive role or suffer dire consequences.

This does not mean that, if he feels that the hospital staff is authoritarian and threatening, he will do everything they want him to do without question or complaint. Not at all! We have learned in the societies of men that the oppressed find all kinds of ways to get back at their oppressors. Of course, the ways that patients find to retaliate against oppression and to reduce somewhat their feelings of powerlessness, often interfere with their getting well. (The patient who does not get well may be viewed, and often is, as their failure by the people who are treating him.) The fact that the patient himself is hurt by his behavior is not so surprising. In all societies people have immolated themselves for similar reasons— from the Buddhist monks of Vietnam who burned themselves alive to protest an oppressive political regime, to the American slaves who often rebelled desperately and futilely against the superior numbers and arms of their owners.

All of this may sound far-fetched to some people. After all, comparing patients to slaves! Really!! But what we must keep in mind is not the *degree* of oppression or frustration but the processes involved in the interaction between authoritarian personnel and people who feel unable to escape from their authority. Even school children with authoritarian teachers respond in similar ways, and are labeled "discipline problems" and "incorrigible" before they are banished to the Siberias of special classes and special schools.

I would conclude, then, that patients are not free as long as they have these fears. One of the questions health personnel must apply themselves to is: "How can we help patients free themselves to take an active part in their own lives while they are in the hospital?"

THE PATIENT
AS A TEAM MEMBER

Most fears generated by authoritarian social situations have, historically, been mitigated when the oppressed people have become full participants in the planning and decision-making that affected their lives. This is the central push of the minority-group movements in the United States today: self-determination, full participation in the decision-making processes, control over those agencies and activities in the community that directly affect their lives.

The principle of self-determination does not, at first, seem applicable to patients. Patients are sick and they need the ministrations of medical experts, not involvement in trial-and-error decision-making processes. Right? Well, let us look at the implications of such a point of view. When poor people say that they want control over the businesses in their area, they are told by government and business experts that they are poor and have no experience in business, so they have no right to make such demands. The consequence is that businesses are established and operated in their neighborhoods that generally take advantage of them and contribute to keeping them poor. The small store overcharges and the chain store sells inferior merchandise. Storekeepers and managers are rude and hostile, and, in addition, take their profits and salaries out of the neighborhood to the more affluent areas where they live and shop. Saloons, liquor stores, factories, and other businesses that contribute to the devaluation of residential areas proliferate. The only people who care feel powerless to do anything to prevent all this.

Here is another example. When Black people talk about community control of police, police authorities are outraged and so are many other people. They insist that "civilians" know nothing about law enforcement and have no right to say how the police—who are experts and professionals —are to do their job. The result of this philosophy has been, especially in cities, that poor Black people see the police as an enemy army. They feel, and often with justification, that policemen harass and mistreat them and violate their rights in ways that white people and middle-class people do not have to endure. To control the police would give them the opportunity to set a policy of fair treatment and to get rid of individuals who act inconsistently with this policy.

There are data that the patient possesses that are vital in planning and executing his health care. He knows how he *feels* about what is being done to him; he knows what his attitude is generally toward illness and being bedridden; he knows what his worries are about his family and his future. These feelings and attitudes can affect how faithfully he follows the doctor's medical orders, how prepared he is psychologically for surgery, how determined he is to get well—all things that the health team needs to know in order to evaluate the effectiveness of its treatment.

If the patient also becomes a part of the health team, then he will develop the freedom to express his feelings and share his ideas just as the other team members do. Just as they become more self-confident, more sure that they are seen as worthwhile in the hospital setting, so the patient does, too. The openness and acceptance reduces the possibility of hidden hostilities and fears and makes the time spent in the hospital salutary, not only for the patient but also for people treating the patient.

HONESTY AND PROFESSIONALISM

Often, the belief that the doctor and the nurse always know what is best for the patient leads to what can only be labeled dishonesty on the part of the professionals. The doctor decides how much he should reveal to the patient about his condition, and the nurse is forced to dissemble and evade the patients' direct questions. Sometimes a family member tells the doctor that the patient should not be informed about some aspect of his illness, and the doctor complies even though he knows little about the family interrelationships and so is unable to evaluate accurately the family member's request. (For example, one woman was expected to spend at least two months in the hospital after a bad accident. The patient's sister told the doctor not to tell the patient, but rather to imply that her stay would be much shorter. The doctor had no way of knowing—nor did he try to find out—that the patient infinitely preferred to know exactly what to expect so that she might delegate her responsibilities and not live from day to day waiting to go back to her regular life.)

Where does honest professional treatment end and dishonesty begin? The answer lies in why we avoid giving a direct answer in a particular situation. Are we really concerned about the danger of retarding the patient's recovery if we tell him the truth? Or are we, perhaps, anticipating an emotional response from the patient and trying to avoid dealing with such a response? Are we also interceding to help the patient's family avoid dealing with the patient's feelings? Is it really for the patient's good that we avoid the truth, or is it more for our own comfort?

And how much of a right does *anyone* have to keep another person in the dark about what is happening to him? Perhaps I go too far in the other direction, but I really don't think anyone has such a right. If an individual prefers not to know about his condition or his treatment, we must leave it to him not to ask about it—or to ask only for what he can handle. Generally, we just do not know other people well enough to make the decision for them.

FEELINGS AND PROFESSIONALISM

There is a myth extant in our society that nurses are tough, that constant exposure to illness, suffering, and death has hardened them and reduced the usual human responsiveness to fellow human beings' pain. So pervasive is this idea that such unresponsiveness is actually believed to be necessary by many nurses. "You're not supposed to get involved," the stricture goes. And the questions many new nurses often ask is, "What can you do when you develop an emotional relationship with a patient and it's necessary to break it off?" and "What can you do to prevent a patient from getting emotionally involved with you?"

It is almost as if nurse-patient relationships are a completely different and unique category of human relationships and that none of the normal rules of people-to-people contact apply. There is also an underlying fear that the nurse—and probably the patient, too—must be protected from the effects of involvement with each other. What effect can be so dangerous as to foster the perpetuation of this caveat? What are we afraid of?

Well, a hospital stay is not a permanent condition of life, so every relationship that develops between a nurse and a patient must soon be terminated. Is it really so necessary to guard ourselves against short-term relationships? We enter upon them very often, do we not? Teachers and students and co-workers do not usually expect life-time friendships to develop among them, but the relatively short time they do have with one another can be satisfying and profitable.

Perhaps part of the feeling of risk involves the inescapable fact that patients are in pain and trouble of some kind and nurses cannot enter upon personal relationships with so many troubled people. Perhaps they feel that their own emotional health cannot survive a larger proportion of empathy and sympathy than most people must have in their relationships.

How accurate is this perception of human relationships? Do not all people have troubles and problems and pain that involve their friends and relations? And are there not many times when friends and relations may share the relief and joy and happiness that enter the lives of patients? Is the emotional commitment to *patients* who are also friends so much different or greater than emotional commitment to other people? Really, I do not think so. I think the pitfall lies in believing that nurses must become involved with all patients or with none at all, when really what we need is an approach to nurse-patient relationships that is not much different from our approach to other human relationships. There are some people for whom we will have great empathy and with whom we may become involved on a very profound level; there are some with whom we will have a rather superficial and casual kind of involvement; and there are some with whom we will have no emotional involvement at all. This is the reality we must expect in all our human relationships.

Nurses, however, have a larger share of responsibility to see to it that no patient is deprived of his share of emotional commitment from *some* member of the health team. Most of the time we go through life making our friends and demonstrating our caring without much regard for the people who are left out, alone, uncared-for. (Remember the girl in high school who never was asked to dance, or the boy whom the girls giggled about and avoided? Engaged as we were in the fierce battle for acceptance, we usually had little time for those who seemed to have lost the battle before we ever got there.) The professional, however, must spend some of his professional energy and expertise in seing to it that *every* patient develops a warm caring relationship with *someone.*

Just another word about expressing feelings. I have never under-stood why it is better to pretend that one has no feelings at seeing someone suffer than it is to cry in sympathy. Surely it goes without saying that the professional—teacher, doctor, or nurse—cannot spend his time crying when he should be working to ameliorate the suffering. There are things he can *do,* so he need not feel quite as frustrated as a non-medical person who cries with frustration and impotence in the face of suffering. But to cry with a sufferer is the human thing to do, and when we deny our feelings we deny our humanity. Eventually, our professional expertise is lessened by such denial, for when we begin to treat diseases rather than people (or teach subjects rather than students) we are simply no longer very good at our jobs.

A FINAL WORD

At some point, we grow very impatient with the constant exploration of issues, the endless participation in simulations, the questioning of experts and the discussing, discussing, discussing—all without coming to clear-cut and absolute conclusions and formulas for effective interaction. The impatience may be understood in terms of a number of factors: (1) Each current generation is steeped in the scientific mystique. The feeling is that if we gather enough data we will inevitably reach predictable conclusions. If we do not know something now, it is just a matter of time before we will know it. (2) Students of nursing have some anxiety about the job they are undertaking, and they are very fearful of making mistakes in situations that are often life-and-death ones. They want to know with some certainty what they may do and what they must not do to get the desired results. (3) Most students who come up in our educational system are accustomed to rely on the authority of the teacher for "correct" answers. An educational setting that offers no correct answers causes some frustration.

Understanding all this, however, does not change the essential facts of human interaction: (1) There are so many variables that despite the knowledge we accumulate, any prediction still inevitably includes a large margin for error. (2) Effective interaction ultimately depends on the skills of the participants in the interaction. Therefore, whatever conclusions we come to about how to interact with others, they must be uniquely our own, and the responsibility for making the most and the best of living in a peopled world is ultimately an individual one. (3) Each one of us is forever developing, forever changing, forever becoming. Although we inevitably make errors in our attempts to sustain human interaction, we need not continue to make the same errors over and over again.